NoBrainer

Nutrition

High energy, flavor filled foods with no cholesterol, low fat and no salt!

Marc Seidman

Published in the United States by Living Health.

ISBN 0-9652015-0-3

Manufactured in the United States of America
Published September 1, 1996

The information in this book reflects the author's experiences and is not intended to replace medical advice. Any questions regarding your health, general or specific, should be addressed to your physician. Before beginning this or any other way of eating consult your physician to be sure it is appropriate for you. The author and publisher expressly disclaim any responsibility for any liability, loss or risk, personal or otherwise which is incurred as a consequence, directly or indirectly, of the use and application of any of the contents of this book.

How to order:

Single copies may be ordered from Living Health at (206) 226-4156. Quantity discounts are available. Fax information concerning the intended use of the books and the number of books you wish to purchase to (206) 226-4023.

This book is printed on acid-free recycled paper to save trees and preserve Earth's ecology.

This book is dedicated to you,
for the opportunity to
share some of my favorite foods♥

May you, your family and friends
be blessed with health and happiness♥

Contents

Acknowledgments

Thanks mom, for preparing fresh, homemade meals. Thanks Jon, for introducing me to the power of the plant kingdom and sharing your foods with me. Thanks family, friends and all those I have shared meals with along the way. May we share many more♥

Thanks Hans, Ayzha, Al, Richard, Shannon, Becky and everyone who helped♥

Thanks Jennifer, for your trust, love and belief in me♥

Introduction

I Love Food...

...the fragrant scents and bursting flavors found in ripe fruit, the mouthwatering smell of garlic and herbs, the warmth of a hearty soup on a cool day , the tempting texture of creamy soups, dressings and sauces, the grain and bean dishes that melt in my mouth, the variety of vivid colors, the creation of tantalizing meals, the sounds of preparing and eating foods...

I feel very fortunate that as I was growing up, my mother prepared homemade meals with quality ingredients. She let me help her around the kitchen. Eating her foods was a joy and spending time with her was very special. My passion for food and health began in mom's kitchen and has flourished since.

I have discovered a way of eating that gives me tremendous energy and makes me look & feel great. I have been eating and enjoying these foods for over 10 years. They are filled with flavor and easy to make. They have no cholesterol, low fat and no salt. I have lost excess fat, gained endurance, built muscle, lowered my cholesterol and have healthier hair, skin & nails.

NoBrainer Nutrition is inspired by Nature's infinite wisdom. All of the nutrients necessary for vibrant health are available from the earth. Mother Nature has made living healthfully simple and fun! I listen to my body... it knows!

NoBrainer Nutrition has simplified my life. I don't think about calories, fat, cholesterol, protein, vitamins, calcium, nutrition... I let Mother Nature take care of that for me. My energy, strength, endurance and medical exams confirm that I am in excellent shape.

NoBrainer Nutrition is my gift to you, your family and friends. Here are some of my favorite foods. May they help make great health and abundant energy part of your life, as well as make eating fun and obtaining optimum nutrition a **"NoBrainer!"**

Marc Seidman

P.S. Read my notes section starting on page 3. I give you some of my secrets, ingredients to stock, useful kitchen appliances & tools, tips, and share with you how to use NoBrainer Nutrition optimally.

NoBrainer
Nutrition

Notes from Marc

I eat 6-8 times throughout the day from morning to early evening. I consider each time I eat a meaningful meal, whether it is a glass of juice, a piece of fruit or a holiday feast.

I have found that eating fruits and their juices in the morning gives me the most energy. In the early afternoon I transition into some of the following: Vegetable juices, soups, salads, sprouts, vegetables, grains, peas & beans, nuts & seeds, pastas, pizzas... I usually end the day with some vegetable juice or herbal tea. You will find the food sections in NoBrainer Nutrition organized the same way.

The meal sizes range from an apple or a glass of juice to a holiday feast. They are alphabetized in their respective section. The recipes are forgiving and adaptable. The amounts of ingredients can be adjusted or altered and you will still be successful. Use common sense. If you want more or less flavor adjust the ingredients.

The serving portions vary and are simplified to give you flexibility and increase your success rate.

In the juice, smoothie, fruit, fruit salad and vegetable sections, use your best judgment. I gave you a rule of thumb for juice and smoothie amounts. Use that to determine how much produce you need to make fresh juice. For fruit, fruit salads, and vegetables ask yourself - How much do I want to eat? Then grab the ingredients and go for it.

The fruit pies can be cut into 6-8 slices. On occasion I have eaten ½ a pie at one sitting. The dried fruit amounts are up to you. The size of salads and sprouts is your choice. The dressings, grains, nuts & seeds, and sauces are designed for 2 servings.

Many of the soups and bean dishes are made in a crockpot. I use a 4 quart version. If I am eating alone I cut the portions in half or have food for the next day. If I am serving 2-4 people there is more than enough.

In addition, I have provided a section for Fun Feasts and Seasonal Menus. Fun Feasts include Holiday, Indian, Italian, Japanese, Mexican, Middle Eastern, and Thai Meals. Seasonal Menus contain 7 days of 8 daily meals from morning until mid evening for the Spring, Summer, Fall and Winter seasons. The 28 different daily menus use foods that are plentiful and in season. At the end of the weekly seasonal menu I include a weekly ingredient list for your shopping convenience.

I provided these menus to give you a guide for creating weekly menus and buying weekly ingredients. Feel free to follow, augment or change them. Most importantly ˙ enjoy what Mother Nature has to offer and let NoBrainer Nutrition empower you!

I love fresh quality ingredients and the freedom of being able to create a sumptuous meal at a moment's notice. Here are some of my secrets:

♦ I visit my favorite produce section once a week and choose whatever is fresh, plentiful and in season. Low prices and abundant availability are great rules of thumb for gathering fresh seasonal foods.

♦ I look for ripe fruits with vibrant colors and fragrant scents. Ripened fruits have more flavor and readily available nutrients.

♦ I collect fresh herbs with rich colors and exhilarating aromas.

♦ Every month or two I buy my dry goods in bulk. I store my beans, grains, nuts, seeds dried herbs, and spices in jars.

The following are samples of the foods I keep in stock and the kitchen appliances and tools I use.

Ingredients to Stock

Beans
Anasazi beans
Black beans
Garbanzo beans
Great northern beans
Kidney beans
Lentils
Lima beans
Navy beans
Pinto beans
Split peas

Grains
Barley
Brown rice(Basmati, long or short grain)
Bulgar (cracked wheat)
Millet

Oats
Quinoa
Wheat(hard winter)

Herbs

Dried
Basil
Cilantro
Cumin
Dill
Garlic
Oregano
Parsley
Thyme

Fresh
Basil
Cilantro
Dill
Garlic
Italian parsley
Oregano
Parsley
Thyme

Nuts & Seeds
Almonds
Cashews
Pine Nuts
Sesame seeds

Pastas
Angel hair
Buckwheat noodles
Fetuccini
Linguini
Penne
Spaghetti
Ziti

Spices
Bragg's
Cayenne
Celery seed
Curry powder
Paprika
Pepper corns
Turmeric
Thai Spices

Others
Arrow root powder
Cinnamon
Maple syrup
Miso
Nori sheets
Olive oil
Popcorn
Wasabi
Water
Whole wheat tortillas

Kitchen Appliances & Tools

Apple cutter
Baking sheets
Baskets
Bowls
Blender
Citrus juicer
Colander
Crock pot
Cutting board
Food processor
Garlic press
Grinder (grains & nuts)
Juicer
Measuring cups
Mixing bowls
Pepper grinder
Pie dish
Salad spinner
Spatulas
Spice rack
Steamer tray
Storage jars
Strainers
Vegetable peeler
Waffle iron
Wok

Additional tips:

Bragg's liquid aminos adds salt flavor without the salt. The salty flavor is naturally found in soy bean amino acids. I use this in many dishes and dressings for added flavor. Use sparingly. It is concentrated.

Candles are wonderful for relaxing, romantic and memorable meals. They are great for a birthday party and in case your power goes out!

Family & friends add so much to food preparation and eating experiences. Whenever I have an opportunity, I share my food!

Food preparation is an art and can be simple or elaborate. I have fun preparing meals. I love exploring the beauty of food and the vivid colors, contrast and richness they provide. I enjoy designing delicious meals or creating culinary masterpieces. Most of all…I have fun!

I use organic foods whenever possible. Most commercial produce and foods are grown with the use of pesticides and preservatives. Organic foods are grown as close to nature as I can find. Organics have a built in quality check. In order, for organic foods to be good quality, they have to be fresh, ripe and grown with care. If not, they will look and taste terrible. Thank God for Mother Nature!

Ingredient amounts are simplified for two servings where applicable. If you are preparing for 4 people, double the amounts. If you are preparing for yourself, use half the amounts. For juices, smoothies, fruits, fruit salads and salads, be creative and explore what amounts and percentages you like. Most of these foods are versatile. Feel free to make modifications and trust your instincts!

Mushrooms are found in the vegetables section for simplification purposes. My humble apologies to the fungi connoisseurs.

Music creates mood and enhances mealtime.

Serving amounts are figured for two servings unless indicated. See ingredient amounts above.

Spices and the amounts to use can vary depending on the source of spices. Use my amounts to guide you. Use your taste buds to refine, augment and develop new versions.

Substitute water for oil when you want to avoid oil in sautés. You can start most dishes off with water.

The taste of food tends to be more flavorful and enhances as it cools off!

The way I make nutrition a **"NoBrainer"** is by using quality ingredients in a simple convenient and fun way that supports me optimally. The side effects I enjoy are endless energy, consistent endurance and feeling great.

I have given you some of my favorite foods. Have fun. The recipes are friendly and have a wide range of adaptability. Enjoy , share and may you be blessed with **continuous vibrant health!**

Fruit Juices

Fruit juices are an exhilarating food to start the day. They are light and supply my body with quality nutrients which are absorbed quickly and efficiently. Fresh fruit juices are instant fuel, put little stress on my body, taste incredible and give me turbo charged energy. They are fun and simple to make, while being convenient and fast. I am juiced and raring to go, when I start my day with liquid energy...

P.S. Our body is like Earth's surface. It is composed of at least 2/3 water. Fresh juices are flowing with living organic waters and ready to nurture our bodies!

Fruit Juices

Apple
Apple/grape
Apple/pear
Apple/pineapple
Apple/ginger
Cantaloupe
Grape
Grapefruit
Honeydew
Melon
Orange
Papaya
Peach
Pear
Pineapple
Tangerine
Tomato
Watermelon

Juice fruit of your choice with a juicer and savor some of Nature's greatest flavors!

A good rule of thumb for juice quantities is, for every 16 ounces of juice you want to make, use about 2 pounds of fruit.

Vegetable Juices

Vegetable juices are a fantastic stabilizer, builder and energizer. They are filled with essential nutrients and help build, balance and restore my body. They augment and enhance my afternoon and evening meals. Vegetable juices are great on their own or before salads, sprouts, soups, vegetables, grains, pastas, pizzas...

P.S. Our body is like Earth's surface. It is composed of at least 2/3 water. Fresh juices are flowing with living organic waters and ready to nurture our bodies!

Vegetable Juices

Carrot

Carrot/apple

Carrot/celery

> **Carrot Juice** has the necessary nutrients to sustain life. It invigorates, heals and is a great base for most vegetable juices.

Carrot/celery/beet

Carrot/celery/beet/parsley

Carrot/celery/lettuce

Carrot/spinach

Carrot/lettuce(romaine)

> **Garlic and Ginger** can be added to any of these vegetable drinks for spicy flavor.

Carrot/cucumber/celery

Carrot/cucumber/celery/beet

Carrot/cucumber/celery/beet/parsley

Celery

Celery/cucumber

Celery/cucumber/lettuce

Celery/cucumber/lettuce/parsley

Cucumber

Lettuce

Juice vegetables of your choice with a juicer and savor some of Nature's greatest flavors!

A good rule of thumb for juice quantities is, for every 16 ounces of juice you want to make, use about 2 pounds of vegetables.

Smoothies & Shakes

Smoothies and shakes are quick, filling and power packed with nutrients. On hot days I am refreshed with frozen smoothies (shakes). Most of the time I savor my smoothies at room or refrigerated temperature. I throw some fresh fruit in a blender with water or juice and whip up a heavenly delight. Smoothies and shakes are more concentrated than fruit juices and tend to give me more continuous energy.

Smoothies & Shakes

Apple/banana
Apple/banana/date
Apple/blueberry
Apple/mango
Apple/papaya
Apple/peach
Apple/pear
Apple/raspberry
Apple/strawberry
Coconut/banana
Coconut/papaya
Orange/mango
Orange/papaya
Orange/peach
Orange/raspberry
Orange/strawberry
Pear/banana
Pineapple/papaya
Pineapple/peach
Pineapple/pear
Pineapple/strawberry

For every 16 ounce smoothie, use between 4-8 ounces of juice and 8-12 ounces of fruit. Blend and serve!

Tip: Sometimes I add dates to my banana smoothie for an extra jolt of energy!

Fruit

Fruit is an ideal food. It is rich in essential nutrients and flowing with living water. I eat raw, ripe fruit which is filled with natural living enzymes. My body is fueled almost immediately and spends little energy on digestion. I feel alive and have abundant energy.

Apples

Apple Chunks with Raisins

Apples
Raisins and/or dates

Peel and core apples. Cut into chunks. Mix with raisins and/or cut up dates. Serve in your favorite bowl.

Apple Sauce

Apples

Peel and core apples. Purée to desired texture in a food processor. Cinnamon is optional.

Shredded Apples with Cinnamon

Apples
Cinnamon

Peel and core apples. Shred with hand shredder or food processor. Sprinkle and mix cinnamon to taste.

Whole Apples

Apples

Wash whole apples and enjoy for snacks or when you are on the run...

Apples come in many varieties. Most apples come from Washington state. They are harvested in the fall, with some in late summer & early winter. Then they are kept in cold storage and shipped out during the year. The best quality and prices can be found between late fall and late winter.

Apricots

Apricots a lá carte!(rinse and serve!)

Apricot Purée

Apricots

Wash apricots and remove pits. Purée in food processor.

Avocados

Avocado Chunks with Apple

Avocado
Apple

Cut avocado in half the long way. Remove pit. Scoop avocado halves out with a spoon. Cut avocado halves into chunks. Peel, core and shred or dice apple. Mix together and serve.

Avocado Chunks with Banana

Avocado
Banana

Cut avocado in half the long way. Remove pit. Scoop avocado halves out with a spoon. Cut avocado into chunks, slice banana, mix together and serve.

Avocado Chunks with Pineapple

Avocado
Pineapple

Cut avocado in half the long way. Remove pit. Scoop avocado halves out with a spoon. Cut avocado halves into chunks. Peel, core and cut pineapple into chunks. Mix avocado and pineapple and serve.

Avocado Dip

1-2 avocados
½ spinach or lettuce
¼ onion
2-4 garlic cloves
1 handful of fresh
chopped herbs like
basil, cilantro, parsley,
dill, thyme(optional)
Fresh ground pepper to taste
Bragg's to taste

Keep dip fresh until it is served by putting the whole avocado pit in the dip and placing it in the refrigerator. When you are ready to serve, remove the pit! This works for a few hours and some times until the next morning.

Cut avocado in half the long way. Remove pit. Scoop avocado halves out with a spoon. Rinse and dry spinach or lettuce in a salad spinner. Finely chop onions, garlic and herbs in a food processor. Add spinach or lettuce to food processor and finely chop. Add avocado halves and blend to desired consistency.

Avocado and Mango

Avocado
Mango

Cut avocado in half the long way. Remove pit. Scoop avocado halves out with a spoon and cut into chunks. Peel and cut mango into chunks. Mix avocado and mango chunks. You are ready to serve.

Avocado Sliced with Cucumber

Avocado
Cucumber

Cut avocado in half the long way. Remove pit. Scoop avocado halves out with a spoon. Slice avocado halves long or short way (your choice, just have fun!). Peel, slice and serve cucumber with avocado.

Avocado Sliced with Tomatoes

Avocado
Tomatoes

Cut avocado in half the long way. Remove pit. Scoop avocado halves out with a spoon. Slice avocado halves long or short way (your choice, just have fun!). Place over round tomato slices. Season or eat plain.

Guacamole

1-2 avocados
¼ onion
2-4 garlic cloves
1 handful of fresh chopped herbs like basil, cilantro, parsley, dill, thyme(optional)
Fresh ground pepper to taste
Bragg's to taste
Lemon, cayenne and ½-1 jalepeño are optional

> **Keep guacamole fresh** until it is served by putting the whole avocado pit in the dip and placing it in the refrigerator. When you are ready to serve, remove the pit! This has worked for a few hours and on some occasions until the next morning.

Cut avocado in half the long way. Remove pit. Scoop avocado halves out with a spoon. Finely chop onion, garlic, jalepeño and herbs in a food processor. Add avocado halves and juice from lemon and blend to desired consistency.

Bananas

Banana Ice Cream

Bananas
With any or all of the following fruits:
(apples, blueberries, coconut, dates, peaches, raisins...)

> **Remember to peel the bananas.** Once I told a man in the gym about these frozen delights. When I asked him if he liked the shake, he was less than enthused. He froze the whole banana. That explained everything!

When brown spots appear, peel bananas and freeze in sealed container Run frozen bananas through champion juicer with blank "screen".

Bananas Puréed with Fruits

Bananas
Your choice of:
(apple, pear, mango, papaya, peaches, nectarines or apricots!)

Purée bananas with fruit in food processor. Great for babies and small children.

Banana Smoothies & Shakes

(See Smoothies & Shakes)

Bananas
Your choice of:
(apple, grape, pear, coconut, papaya, peach...)

Whole Bananas

Bananas

Peel and eat when brown spots appear for optimum ripeness and nutrition.

Blackberries

Blackberries a lá carte!

Rinse blackberries and serve!

Blackberry Fruit Salad

Blackberries
Raspberries
Strawberries

Mix berries and serve.

Blueberries

Blueberries a lá carte!

Blueberries with Peaches

Blueberries
Peaches

Rinse blueberries. Peel, remove pits and slice peaches. Mix blueberries and peaches. You're ready to eat.

Cantaloupe

Cantaloupe Chunks

Cantaloupe

Cut cantaloupe in half. Remove seeds and skin. Cut into chunks and serve.

Cantaloupe Halves or Wedges

Cantaloupe

Cut cantaloupe in half and remove seeds. Serve with a spoon. If you prefer wedges cut into wedges and serve.

Melon Salad

Cantaloupe
Honeydew
Watermelon
Melons of your choice (optional)

Cut cantaloupe, honeydew, watermelon and any other of your favorite melons into chunks. Mix in a bowl and serve.

Cherries

Cherries a lá carte!

Cranberries

Cranberry Juice

Cranberries

Rinse and juice on their own or with apples.

Cranberry Sauce

8-12 ounces cranberries
4-6 ounces apple juice
¼ orange

Rinse cranberries and bring to a boil in apple juice with an orange quarter (including peel). Turn heat down to simmer for 5-10 minutes. Remove from heat and let cool to room temperature. Place in refrigerator to cool and firm up.

Dates

Coconut Apple Date Balls

½ coconut
1 apple
8-10 dates
1-2 tablespoons carob powder (optional)

Remove coconut from shell and pits from dates. Core and peel apples. Shred coconut in food processor. Add pitted dates and blend into a chunky paste. Then blend in peeled and cored apples. Mix in optional carob powder. Remove paste from food processor, mix, form into balls and chill in refrigerator until firm (20-30 minutes).

Coconut Date Balls

½ coconut
8-10 dates

Remove coconut from shell and pits from dates. Shred coconut in food processor. Add pitted dates and blend into a chunky paste. Remove paste from food processor, mix, form into balls and chill in refrigerator until firm (20-30 minutes).

No Bake Pie Crust

1 coconut
15-20 dates

Food processor preparation

Remove coconut from shell and pits from dates. Shred coconut in food processor. Add pitted dates and blend into a chunky paste. Remove paste from food processor, mix, form into crust in pie dish. Chill in refrigerator until firm (20-30 minutes).

Champion juicer preparation

Remove coconut from shell and pits from dates. Run pitted dates followed by coconut through champion juicer with blank "screen". Mix date paste and shredded coconut to form a crust in a pie shell. Then chill in refrigerator until firm (20-30 minutes).

Quick Pick Me Up

Dates a lá carte!

Figs

Figs a lá carte!

Grapes

Grapes a lá carte!

Rinse grapes,
remove from stem and eat!

> **Try freezing grapes**
> and eating them for a
> refreshing snack.
> **They are Delicious!**

Grapefruit

Citrus salad (see Fruit Salads)

Grapefruit Chunks or Halves

Grapefruit

Peel grapefruit and cut into chunks or cut grapefruit in half (parallel to where the skin was attached to the tree) and serve.

Lemons & Limes

Use in citrus punch, dressings, over salad and with avocado or asparagus.

Mangos

Mango a lá carte!, chunks, salad, slices...

Olives

Use in bread, on pizza and in salads...

Oranges

Citrus salad (see Fruit Salads)

Oranges a lá carte!

Papayas

Papaya a lá carte!, chunks, salad, slices...

Papaya

Cut papaya in half, remove seeds, serve and eat.

Peaches

Peaches a lá carte!, juice, pie, puréed, slices...

Rinse peaches and serve!

Pears

Pears a lá carte!, fruit salads, juice, puréed, slices...

Rinse pears and serve!

Pineapples

Chunks, fruit salads, juice, slices...

Plums

Juice, whole...

Raspberries

Raspberries a lá carte!, fruit salads, smoothies & shakes...

Strawberries

Strawberries a lá carte, frozen, fruit salads, juices, smoothies & shakes...

Tomatoes

Whole, slices, wedges, soups, salsa, dressings, sauces...

Fruit Salads

When I make fruit salads, I feel like I am creating a piece of art... vibrant colors, bursting flavors and tantalizing textures to savor and enjoy! Fruit salads are refreshing and full of instant energy. They are fun, quick and convenient. Here are some of my favorites...

Apple, Pear, Banana, Raisin Fruit Salad

Apple
Pear
Banana
Raisins

Peel (Peeling is optional. If you want the skin, skip the peeling.) apple and pear. Remove core and cut into chunks. Peel and slice banana. Mix apple chunks, pear chunks, banana slices and raisins in a dish and serve.

Apple, Pear, Peach, Banana, Papaya, Raisin Fruit Salad

Apple
Pear
Peach
Banana
Papaya
Raisin

Peel (Peeling is optional. If you want the skin, skip the peeling.) apple and pear. Remove core and cut into chunks. Cut peach in half, remove pit, peel and cut into chunks. Peel and slice banana. Cut papaya in half and remove seeds. Peel papaya and cut into chunks. Mix apple, pear, peach and papaya chunks with banana slices and raisins in a dish and serve.

Avocado, Peach, Banana, Blueberry Fruit Salad

Avocado
Peach
Banana
Blueberry

Cut avocado in half the long way. Remove pit. Scoop avocado halves out with a spoon. Cut avocado into chunks. Cut peach in half, remove pits, peel and cut into chunks. Peel and slice banana. Rinse blueberries and dry on a paper or cloth towel. Mix avocado and peach chunks with banana slices and rinsed blueberries in a dish and serve.

Banana, Date, Coconut Fruit Salad

Banana
Dates
Coconut

Peel and slice banana. Remove date pits and cut into pieces. Shred coconut. Mix banana slices with date pieces in a dish and sprinkle shredded coconut on top and serve.

Melon Salad

Cantaloupe
Honey dew
Watermelon

Peel cantaloupe and honeydew, remove seeds and cut into chunks. Remove watermelon from rind and cut into chunks. Mix cantaloupe, honeydew and watermelon chunks in a dish and serve.

Orange, Grapefruit, Pineapple Fruit Salad

Orange
Grapefruit
Pineapple

Peel orange and grapefruit and cut into bite size pieces. Peel pineapple remove the core and cut into chunks. Mix orange and grapefruit pieces with pineapple chunks in a dish and serve.

Papaya, Banana, Raisin Fruit Salad

Papaya
Banana
Raisin or currant

Cut papaya in half and remove seeds. Peel papaya and cut into chunks. Peel and slice banana. Mix banana slices and papaya chunks with raisins or currants in a dish and serve.

Papaya, Mango, Banana Fruit Salad

Papaya
Mango
Banana

Cut papaya in half and remove seeds. Peel papaya and cut into chunks. Peel mango, remove seed and cut into chunks. Peel and slice banana. Mix papaya, mango and banana chunks in a dish and serve.

Papaya, Pineapple, Avocado Fruit Salad

Papaya
Pineapple
Avocado

Cut papaya in half and remove seeds. Peel papaya and cut into chunks. Peel pineapple remove the core and cut into chunks. Cut avocado in half the long way. Remove pit. Scoop avocado halves out with a spoon. Cut avocado into chunks. Mix papaya, pineapple and avocado chunks in a dish and serve.

Papaya, Pineapple, Strawberry Fruit Salad

Papaya
Pineapple
Strawberry

Cut papaya in half and remove seeds. Peel papaya and cut into chunks. Peel pineapple remove the core and cut into chunks. Rinse strawberries and cut into halves or quarters. Mix papaya and pineapple chunks with strawberry pieces in a dish and serve.

Peach, Blueberry Fruit Salad

Peach
Blueberry

Cut peaches in half, remove pits, peel and cut into chunks. Rinse blue berries and dry on a paper towel. Mix peach chunks and rinsed blueberries in a dish and serve.

Dried Fruit

Dried fruit is quick, convenient and bursting with vital nutrients. It is condensed, concentrated, compact and lightweight. I take dried fruit on hikes, climbing, snow skiing and almost anywhere I can use some instantaneous, sustainable energy. Also, on occasion I reconstitute dried fruit with water. I add water to the dried fruit and let it soften. Then I blend it into a purée or fruit soup with fresh slices of bananas.

Dried Fruit

Apples
Apricots
Bananas
Cherries
Dates
Figs (Black Mission) - soup with banana slices
Figs (Calimyrna)
Mangos
Mulberries
Papaya
Peaches
Pears
Pineapple
Prunes
Raisins

Eat dried fruits on their own, or reconstitute with water. Add water to the dried fruit until it softens (10-20 minutes). Then blend it into a purée or fruit soup with fresh chunks of fruit. One of my favorites is fig soup with banana slices.

Fruit Pies

Fruit pies are awesome. They tantalize my taste buds. They make my tongue dance and my lips sing. They make me feel good all over. When I have some extra time and feel like "wowing" someone special I whip up a raw fruit pie.

No Bake Pie Crust

1 coconut
15-20 dates

Food processor preparation

Remove coconut from shell and pits from dates. Shred coconut in food processor. Add pitted dates and blend into a chunky paste. Remove paste from food processor, mix, form into crust in pie dish and chill in refrigerator to firm (20-30 minutes).

Champion juicer preparation

Remove coconut from shell and pits from dates. Run pitted dates followed by coconut through champion juicer with blank. Mix date paste and shredded coconut to form a crust in a pie shell. Then chill in refrigerator to firm (20-30 minutes).

Apple Pie

15 dates
1 coconut
4 apples
Cinnamon (optional)

Make no bake pie crust. Shred apples and mix with cinnamon. Pour into crust and you're done!

Apple/Pear Pie

15 dates
1 coconut
2 apples
2 pears
Cinnamon (optional)

Make no bake pie crust. Peel, core and shred apples. Mix with cinnamon. Peel, core and slice pears. Alternate four layers of apples, and pear slices in crust. Start with apples. Chill and serve.

Banana Coconut Cream Pie

8 bananas
20 dates
1 coconut

Make no bake pie crust. Save one tablespoon of shredded coconut for topping. Mix two tablespoons of date paste (from crust mixture) with two bananas into a thick, creamy consistency. Slice 2 bananas into the pie crust to make one layer of bananas. Then pour some of the cream mixture on top, add another layer of 2 bananas, add the rest of the cream, and another layer of 2 bananas. Sprinkle shredded coconut on top of pie and refrigerate until firm. (1/2 hr if you can wait!)

Mango Pie

15 dates
1 coconut
3-5 mangos

Make no bake pie crust. Peel and slice mangos. Layer mangos in pie crust. Chill and serve.

Papaya Pie

15 dates
1 coconut
2 pounds of papaya flesh

Make no bake pie crust mentioned above. Peel, seed and slice papaya. Layer papaya in pie crust. Chill and serve.

Peach Pie

15 dates
1 coconut
4-5 peaches

Make no bake pie crust mentioned above.   Peel, remove pits and slice peaches. Layer peaches in pie crust. Chill and serve.

Peach/Blueberry Pie

20 dates
1 coconut
3 peaches
½ pint of blueberries

Make no bake pie crust mentioned above.   Make blueberry date paste by mix two tablespoons of date paste (from crust mixture) with blueberries into a thick paste. Peel, remove pits and slice peaches. Layer peaches, blueberry spread, peaches, blueberry spread, peaches in pie crust. Chill and serve.

Salads

Salads are convenient, simple and fun to make. They are flowing with living waters, rich colors and provide me with vital nutrients. Vegetables become artistic creations bursting with flavor for my palate to savor. Salads served in a large bowl with a creamy dressing are one of my favorite meals.

Asparagus Salad

Steamed or uncooked asparagus served over bib or butter lettuce with a lemon herb dressing.

Asparagus
Bib or butter lettuce
Pepper
Lemon herb dressing

> **Asparagus bottoms** tend to be hard and filled with fiber. Either peel the bottoms with a vegetable peeler or cut them off (approximately 1 inch).

Rinse lettuce and spin dry in a salad spinner. Wash asparagus and steam until desired texture. Serve asparagus over lettuce with lemon herb dressing.

Avocado Salad

Avocado chunks with tomato, onion and garlic.

Avocado
Tomato
Onion
Garlic
Dill
Pepper
Lemon
Sprouts and/or lettuce

Cut avocado in half long way, remove pit, and scoop out with a spoon. Cut avocado, tomato, onion into chunks. Mix with chopped dill, pressed garlic, squeezed lemon juice and fresh pepper. Serve over sprouts and/or lettuce. Top with a small piece of dill or parsley for flair.

Cabbage Salad

Finely shredded cabbage with tomato and lemon herb dressing.

Cabbage
Tomato
Lemon herb dressing

Chop or shred cabbage finely in a food processor. Then mix with diced tomatoes and lemon herb dressing.

Cauliflower Salad

Chopped cauliflower with tomato and lemon herb dressing.

Cauliflower
Tomato
Onion (optional)
Parsley
Lemon herb dressing

Chop cauliflower. Dice onions. Cut tomatoes into chunks. Then mix with lemon herb dressing and serve.

Cucumber Salads

Cucumber and Avocado Salad

Cucumber
Avocado
Dill
Bragg's

Cut avocado in half long way, remove pit, and scoop out with a spoon. Cut avocado, and peeled cucumber into chunks. Mix with chopped dill, Bragg's and pepper.

Cucumber and Tomato Salad

Cucumber
Tomato
Onion
Dill
Lemon
Fresh ground pepper
Bragg's to taste

Cut tomato, onion and peeled cucumber into chunks. Mix with finely chopped dill, lemon, Bragg's and fresh ground pepper.

Curried Cucumber Salad 1

Cucumber
Onion
Garlic
Curry spices

Peel, cut in half at the center and slice cucumber halves lengthwise into thin strips. Slice onion and mix with curry spices and pressed garlic.

Curried Cucumber Salad 2

Shred cucumber and onion with manual shredder or food processor. Then mix with curry spices and pressed garlic.

Spicy Thai Cucumber Salad 1

Cucumber
Onion
Garlic
Thai spices
Lemon (optional)

Peel, cut in half at the center and slice cucumber halves lengthwise into thin strips. Slice onion and mix with Thai spices and pressed garlic.

Spicy Thai Cucumber Salad 2

Shred cucumber and onion with manual shredder or food processor. Then mix with Thai spices and pressed garlic.

Garden Salads

Colorful Garden Salad

Romaine
Sprouts
Cucumber
Tomato
Corn
Scallions or onion
Herbs
Pepper

> **Salad spinners** are great for removing water from rinsed greens.

Clean lettuce and spin dry in a salad spinner. Cut up lettuce and place in serving bowl, or on a plate. Cover lettuce with sprouts. Then place tomato chunks, wedges or slices over sprouts. Cover tomato with corn. Then sprinkle fresh chopped herbs and scallions on top of the corn. Serve with your favorite dressing and fresh ground pepper.

Miso Garden Salad

Romaine
Sprouts
Shredded carrots
Shredded beats
Shredded daikon
Miso dressing

Clean lettuce and spin dry in a salad spinner. Cut up lettuce and place in serving bowl or on a plate. Cover lettuce with sprouts. Then separately place shredded carrots, beets and daikon next to each other over sprouts. Serve with miso dressing and fresh ground pepper.

Avocado Garden Salad

Romaine
Tomato
Cucumber
Scallions or onion
Avocado
Herbs

Clean lettuce and spin dry in a salad spinner. Cut up lettuce and place in serving bowl or on a plate. Then place tomato chunks, wedges or slices over lettuce. Cover tomato with peeled and diced cucumber. Top cucumber with diced or sliced avocado. Then sprinkle fresh chopped herbs and scallions or onion on top. Serve with your favorite dressing and fresh ground pepper.

Italian Salad

Arugala, endive, radicchio and watercress served with extra virgin olive oil, balsamic vinegar and fresh pepper. You can substitute lemon for the vinegar.

Arugala
Endive
Radicchio
Watercress
Extra virgin olive oil
Balsamic vinegar or lemon
Fresh ground pepper
Bragg's to taste

Clean and spin dry arugala, endive, radicchio and watercress. Then display leaves of each next to each other. Serve with olive oil, balsamic vinegar Bragg's and fresh ground pepper.

Mexican Salad

Shredded lettuce
Sprouts
Black beans **(see Peas & Beans)**
Avocado
Scallions or onion
Fresh ground pepper to taste
Bragg's to taste

Shred lettuce of your choice in food processor. Top with sprouts. Cover with beans. Put chunks of avocado over beans and top off with chopped scallions or onion.

Pepper Salad

Red, green & yellow peppers
Onion (optional)
Extra virgin olive oil
Balsamic vinegar or lemon
Fresh ground pepper to taste
Bragg's to taste

Wash and dry peppers. Slice or chunk peppers and onion. Serve with olive oil, balsamic vinegar and fresh ground pepper.

Romaine Salad

Romaine with creamy garlic or Caesar dressing.

Romaine
Creamy garlic or Caesar dressing
Pepper

Clean lettuce and spin dry in a salad spinner. Cut up lettuce and place in serving bowl, on a plate or in a bowl. Serve with creamy garlic or Caesar dressing and fresh ground pepper.

Spinach Salad

Spinach
Sprouts
Tomato
Onion
Avocado (optional)

Clean spinach and spin dry in a salad spinner. Cut up spinach and place in serving bowl, on a plate or in a bowl. Cover spinach with sprouts. Then place tomato chunks, wedges or slices over sprouts. Cover tomato with avocado slices or chunks. Serve with your favorite dressing and fresh ground pepper.

Spinach/Mushroom Salad

Spinach and sliced mushrooms served with lemon herb dressing. **(Follow the instructions above).**

Sprout Salad

Buckwheat sprouts
Sunflower sprouts
Pea greens
Alfalfa or clover sprouts
Italian or lemon herb dressing

Clean greens and spin dry in a salad spinner. Place greens in serving bowl or on a plate. Cover greens with sprouts. Serve with Italian or lemon herb dressing and fresh ground pepper.

Tomato Salad

Tomato, onion and dill with lemon herb or Italian dressing.

Tomatoes
Onion
Dill
Pepper
Garlic
Lemon herb or Italian dressing

Slice or chunk tomatoes. Cover tomatoes with chopped dill, pressed garlic and onion. Serve with lemon herb or Italian dressing and fresh ground pepper.

Vegetable Salad

Steamed vegetables (asparagus, broccoli, carrots cauliflower, garlic, onion, yellow squash, zucchini...)
Bib or butter lettuce

Chill steamed vegetables and mix with Italian or lemon herb dressing. Serve over chopped bib or butter lettuce.

Sprouts

Sprouts are alive and full of vital enzymes, vitamins, minerals and nutrients. Sprouts come from germinated grains, nuts, seeds and legumes. Water is added to these hibernating foods. They are awakened and continue the cycle of life. Dry, raw grains, nuts, seeds and legumes soaked in water break down their fat, protein and carbohydrates into fuel for growth. This sprouting process jump starts the foods and prepares them for photosynthesis. Sprouts are power foods! They add tremendous value to juices, salads, roll ups, grain dishes, hummous, or avocados.

Sprouts

Alfalfa
Bean
Buckwheat
Clover
Fenugreek
Lentil
Pea
Radish
Sunflower

Sprouts are great with salads, on their own, in juices in roll ups, with grains, hummous and avocados!

Dressings

Dressings are filled with life, energy and robust flavor. I pack them full of fresh herbs, spices and sumptuous ingredients. They are simple and easy to make, while being quick and convenient. Most of all they make salads, vegetables and sprouts taste incredible!

Avocado Dressing

1 avocado
½ peeled lemon (optional)
½-1 clove garlic
¼ cup chopped parsley
1 teaspoon fresh thyme or oregano leaves
A few basil leaves and other herbs (optional)
Fresh ground pepper to taste
Bragg's to taste
4-8 ounces of water for desired thickness

Remove seeds from lemon. Put ingredients into a blender. Blend until desired creamy consistency. You're ready to use.

Avocado Tomato Basil Dressing

1 avocado
8-16 ounces of tomato for desired thickness
½ peeled lemon(optional)
1-2 garlic cloves
¼ cup chopped parsley
1 teaspoon thyme or oregano leaves
A few basil leaves and other herbs (optional)
Fresh ground pepper to taste
Bragg's to taste

> **Dressing can be distributed evenly** by covering your salads in layers as you add more ingredients.

Remove seeds from lemon. Put ingredients into a blender. Blend until desired creamy consistency. You're ready to use.

Caesar Dressing

½-1 lemon (juice)
1-2 garlic cloves
4-6 ounces soaked cashews
2-4 ounces water from soaked cashews for
desired consistency
Fresh ground pepper to taste
Bragg's to taste

Put ingredients in a blender. Blend until desired creamy consistency.
You're ready to use.

Creamy Dill Dressing

¼ cup fresh dill or ½ teaspoon dried dill
1-2 garlic cloves
4-6 ounces soaked cashews
2-4 ounces water from soaked cashews for
desired consistency
Fresh ground pepper to taste
Bragg's to taste

Put ingredients into a blender. Blend until desired creamy consistency.
You're ready to use.

Creamy Garlic Dressing

1-2 garlic cloves
4-6 ounces soaked cashews
2-4 ounces water from soaked
cashews for desired consistency
Fresh ground pepper to taste
Bragg's to taste

Paprika can be used for its robust color to decorate light colored sauces and foods. Sprinkle on top of sauce or food before you serve.

Put ingredients into a blender. Blend until desired creamy consistency.
You're ready to use.

Italian Dressing

1-2 garlic cloves
½ peeled lemon or 1-2 ounces balsamic vinegar
¼ cup chopped cilantro
¼ cup chopped parsley
1 teaspoon thyme or oregano leaves
A few basil leaves and other herbs (optional)
1 tablespoon olive oil
4-8 ounces water for desired consistency
Fresh ground pepper to taste
Bragg's to taste

Remove seeds from lemon. Put ingredients into a blender. Blend, you're ready to use.

Lemon Dill Dressing

1-2 garlic cloves
½ peeled lemon
¼ cup chopped dill
A few basil leaves and other herbs (optional)
1 tablespoon olive oil
4-8 ounces water for desired consistency
Fresh ground pepper to taste
Bragg's to taste

Remove seeds from lemon. Put ingredients into a blender. Blend, you're ready to use.

Lemon Herb Dressing

1-2 garlic cloves
½ peeled lemon
¼ cup chopped cilantro
¼ cup chopped parsley
1 teaspoon thyme or oregano leaves
A few basil leaves and other herbs (optional)
1 tablespoon olive oil
4-8 ounces water for desired consistency
Fresh ground pepper to taste
Bragg's to taste

Remove seeds from lemon. Put ingredients into a blender. Blend, you're ready to use.

Miso Dressing

1-2 garlic cloves
2-3 tablespoons of sweet mellow miso
¼ cup chopped cilantro
¼ cup chopped parsley
1 teaspoon thyme or oregano leaves
A few basil leaves and other herbs (optional)
1 tablespoon olive oil
4-8 ounces water for desired consistency
Fresh ground pepper to taste
Bragg's to taste

Put ingredients into a blender. Blend, you're ready to use.

Olive Oil and Lemon or Balsamic Vinegar

Olive oil
Balsamic vinegar or lemon
Fresh ground pepper

Pour over salad and eat.

> **I use cold pressed raw olive oil whenever it is available.**

Tahini Dressing

1-2 garlic cloves
4-6 ounces soaked sesame seeds
½ teaspoon cumin powder
¼ teaspoon paprika
Fresh ground pepper to taste
Bragg's to taste

Put ingredients into a blender. Blend, you're ready to use.

Tomato Basil Dressing

16 ounces of tomatoes
½ peeled lemon (optional)
1-2 garlic cloves
¼ cup chopped parsley
1 teaspoon thyme or oregano leaves
A few leaves of basil and other herbs (optional)
Fresh ground pepper to taste
Bragg's to taste

Remove seeds from lemon. Put ingredients into a blender. Blend, you're ready to use.

Soups

Uncooked

Uncooked soups can be whipped up in less than 5 minutes with a blender or a food processor. They are wonderful on a warm day. They are refreshing, invigorating and taste great.

Cooked

Cooked soups can take from 20 minutes to 12 hours. Most of them take under 15 minutes to prepare and serve. The rest of the time is spent cooking. These soups are soothing and comfortably filling and are great with a salad.

Uncooked Soups

Avocado Soup

1 avocado
½ peeled lemon (optional)
½-1 garlic cloves
¼ cup chopped parsley
1 teaspoon of thyme or oregano
A few basil leaves and other herbs (optional)
Fresh ground pepper to taste
Bragg's to taste
8-12 ounces water for desired thickness

Remove seeds from lemon. Put ingredients into a blender or food processor. Blend, you're ready to serve.

Corn Soup

2-4 ears corn
¼ cup chopped lemon basil
½ garlic cloves
Fresh ground pepper to taste
Bragg's to taste
4-8 ounces water for desired consistency

Put ingredients into a blender or food processor. Blend, you're ready to serve.

Gazpacho Soup

1 pepper
1 cucumber
1 tomato
½ onion
½ peeled lemon (optional)
1-2 garlic cloves
¼ cup chopped parsley
1 teaspoon thyme or oregano
A few basil leaves and other herbs (optional)
Fresh ground pepper to taste
Bragg's to taste

Remove lemon seeds. Dice up onions, peppers, tomatoes and cucumbers. Mix together with garlic, herbs and spices. You're ready to serve.

Tomato Soup

Avocado chunks
16 ounces tomatoes
½ peeled lemon (optional)
1-2 garlic cloves
¼ cup chopped parsley
1 teaspoon thyme or oregano leaves
A few basil leaves and other herbs (optional)
Fresh ground pepper to taste
Bragg's to taste

Remove lemon seeds. Put ingredients into a blender or food processor. Blend and add avocado chunks to bowl, you're ready to serve.

Cooked Soups

Anasazi Bean Soup

16 ounces soaked anasazi beans
1-2 peppers (red, yellow or green)
1 onion
4-8 garlic cloves
¼ cup chopped cilantro
¼ cup chopped parsley
1 teaspoon thyme or oregano leaves
¼ cup basil and other herbs (optional)
2-4 cups water for desired consistency
Fresh ground pepper to taste
Bragg's to taste

Soak beans with 3 times as much water overnight for 8 hours. In the morning chop or dice ingredients and add to crockpot with water on high. In 8 hours your meal is ready to be served. For added color add ¼ cup chopped peppers to bowl of soup. If you want a creamy soup, blend in blender or food processor.

Asparagus Soup

½-1 bunch asparagus (16-24 ounces)
½ garlic clove
4-8 ounces water for desired consistency
Fresh ground pepper to taste
Bragg's to taste

Steam asparagus until tender. Put ingredients in blender or food processor. Blend, you're ready to serve.

Barley Soup

12 ounces soaked barley
2-4 carrots
2-3 stems celery
8 ounces mushrooms
1 onion
4-8 garlic cloves
¼ cup dill
¼ cup chopped parsley
1 teaspoon thyme or oregano leaves
4-6 cups water for desired consistency
Fresh ground pepper to taste
Bragg's to taste

Soak barley overnight for 8 hours. In the morning chop or dice ingredients and add to crockpot with water on high. In 8 hours your meal is ready to be served.

Barley/Split Pea Soup

4 ounces soaked barley
12 ounces soaked split peas
2-4 carrots
2-3 stems celery
8 ounces mushrooms
1 onion
4-8 garlic cloves
¼ cup dill
¼ cup chopped parsley
1 teaspoon thyme or oregano leaves
6-8 cups water for desired consistency
Fresh ground pepper to taste
Bragg's to taste

Soak barley and split peas overnight for 8 hours. In the morning chop or dice ingredients and add to crockpot with water on high. In 8 hours your meal is ready to be served.

Black Bean Soup

16 ounces soaked black beans
1-2 peppers
(red, yellow or green)
1 onion
4-8 garlic cloves
¼ cup cilantro
¼ cup chopped parsley
1 teaspoon thyme or oregano leaves
¼ cup basil and other herbs (optional)
2-4 cups water for desired consistency
Fresh ground pepper to taste
Bragg's to taste

> **Crockpots** can be used to cook most soups and bean dishes. They are very convenient and take little monitoring. They also fill your home with the aroma of a gourmet restaurant.

Soak beans with 3 times as much water overnight for 8 hours. In the morning chop or dice ingredients and add to crockpot with water on high. In 8 hours your meal is ready to be served. For added color add ¼ cup chopped peppers to bowl of soup. If you want a creamy soup, blend in blender or food processor.

Cream of Broccoli Soup

½ broccoli (16-24 ounces)
½ garlic cloves
4-8 ounces water for desired consistency
Fresh ground pepper to taste
Bragg's to taste

Steam broccoli until it is tender. Put ingredients into a blender or food processor. Blend, you're ready to serve.

Cream of Cauliflower Soup

½ cauliflower (16-24 ounces)
½ garlic cloves
4-8 ounces water for desired consistency
Fresh ground pepper to taste
Bragg's to taste

Steam cauliflower until it is tender. Put ingredients into a blender or food processor. Blend, you're ready to serve.

Cream of Corn Soup

3-4 ears corn
½ garlic cloves
2-3 leaves lemon basil
4-8 ounces water for desired consistency
Fresh ground pepper to taste
Bragg's to taste

Steam corn until it is tender. Remove kernels and put ingredients into a blender or food processor. Blend, you're ready to serve.

Creamy Black Bean Soup

16 ounces soaked black beans
1-2 peppers (red, yellow or green)
1 onion
4-8 garlic cloves
¼ cup chopped cilantro and parsley
1 teaspoon thyme or oregano leaves
¼ cup basil and other herbs (optional)
2-4 cups water for desired consistency
Fresh ground pepper to taste
Bragg's to taste

Soak beans overnight for 8 hours. In the morning chop or dice ingredients and add to crockpot with water on high for 8 hours. Purée in food processor or blender. Top with chopped onion if desired and serve.

Creamy Curry Chickpea Soup

16 ounces soaked garbanzo beans
2-3 carrots
1 onion
4-8 garlic cloves
¼ cup chopped parsley
1 teaspoon thyme or oregano leaves
Curry spices
2-4 cups water for desired consistency
Fresh ground pepper to taste
Bragg's to taste

Soak beans overnight for 8 hours. In the morning, chop or dice ingredients and add to crockpot with water on high for 8 hours. Purée in food processor or blender with curry spices, pepper and Bragg's. Then serve.

Garbanzo Bean Soup

16 ounces soaked garbanzo beans
2-3 carrots
1 onion
4-8 garlic cloves
¼ cup chopped parsley
1 teaspoon thyme or oregano leaves
2-4 cups water for desired consistency
Fresh ground pepper to taste
Bragg's to taste

Soak beans overnight for 8 hours. In the morning, chop or dice ingredients and add to crockpot with water on high for 8 hours. Purée in food processor or blender and serve.

Lentil Soup

16 ounces soaked lentils
2-3 carrots
2-3 stems celery
1 onion
4-8 garlic cloves
¼ cup chopped parsley
1 teaspoon thyme or oregano leaves
2-4 cups water for desired consistency
Fresh ground pepper to taste
Bragg's to taste

Soak lentils overnight for 8 hours. In the morning, chop or dice ingredients and add to crockpot with water on high. In 8 hours your meal is ready to be served.

Lima Bean Soup

16 ounces soaked lima beans
2-3 carrots
2-3 stems celery
1 onion
4-8 garlic cloves
¼ cup chopped parsley
1 teaspoon thyme or oregano leaves
¼ cup basil and other herbs (optional)
2-4 cups water for desired consistency
Fresh ground pepper to taste
Bragg's to taste

Soak lima beans overnight for 8 hours. In the morning, chop or dice ingredients and add to crockpot with water on high. In 8 hours your meal is ready to be served.

Miso Soup

2-3 carrots
2-3 stems celery
1 onion
Vegetables of choice
4-8 garlic cloves
¼ cup chopped parsley
1 teaspoon thyme or oregano
¼ cup basil and other herbs (optional)
2-4 cups water for desired consistency
Fresh ground pepper to taste
Sweet miso to taste

Make your favorite vegetable soup. Fill a pot of water with vegetables like broccoli, carrots, celery, zucchini...Bring to a boil, then simmer for 40-60 minutes.

When soup is finished, pour some of the soup broth into your serving bowl and mix in desired miso (start with 1 teaspoon) until diluted, add vegetables and more broth. You're ready to serve.

Mushroom Soup

16 ounces mushrooms
1 onion
4-8 garlic cloves
1 teaspoon thyme or oregano leaves
¼ cup basil and other herbs (optional)
2-4 cups water for desired consistency
Fresh ground pepper to taste
Bragg's to taste

Put ingredients into pot. Bring to a boil. Then lower temperature of burner to simmer on low for about 40-60 minutes.

Onion Soup

1-2 onions
4-8 garlic cloves
¼ cup chopped parsley
1 teaspoon thyme or oregano
2-4 cups water for desired consistency
Fresh ground pepper to taste
Bragg's to taste

Put ingredients into pot. Bring to a boil. Then lower temperature of burner to simmer on low for about 40-60 minutes.

Potato Soup

3-5 potatoes (1-2 pounds)
2-3 carrots
2-3 stems celery
1 onion
4-8 garlic cloves
¼ cup chopped parsley
1 teaspoon thyme or oregano
¼ cup basil and other herbs (optional)
2-4 cups water for desired consistency
Fresh ground pepper to taste
Bragg's to taste

Put ingredients into pot. Bring to a boil. Then lower temperature of burner to simmer on low for about 40-60 minutes.

Red Lentil Soup

16 ounces soaked red lentils
2-4 carrots
2-3 stems celery
1 onion
4-8 garlic cloves
¼ cup dill
¼ cup chopped parsley
1 tablespoon of leaves thyme or oregano
4-6 cups water for desired consistency
Fresh ground pepper to taste
Bragg's to taste

Soak lentils overnight for 8 hours. In the morning, chop or dice ingredients and add to crockpot with water on high. In 8 hours your meal is ready to be served.

Split Pea Soup

16 ounces soaked split peas
2-4 carrots
2-3 stems celery
1 onion
4-8 garlic cloves
¼ cup dill
¼ cup chopped parsley
1 teaspoon thyme or oregano leaves
4-6 cups water for desired consistency
Fresh ground pepper to taste
Bragg's to taste

Soak split peas overnight for 8 hours. In the morning, chop or dice ingredients and add to crockpot with water on high. In 8 hours your meal is ready to be served.

Vegetable Soup

2-3 carrots
2-3 stems celery
1 onion
Vegetables of choice
4-8 garlic cloves
¼ cup chopped parsley
1 teaspoon thyme or oregano leaves
¼ cup chopped basil leaves and other herbs (optional)
2-4 cups water for desired consistency
Fresh ground pepper to taste
Bragg's to taste

Make your favorite vegetable soup. Fill a pot of water with vegetables like broccoli, carrots, celery, zucchini... Bring to a boil, then simmer for 40-60 minutes. If you want to spice up your soup, try adding cayenne, Thai spices, curry spices or hot peppers to desired taste. Also, you can purée this soup in a blender or food processor. Sometimes I have it chunky and sometimes I have it creamy.

Vegetables

Vegetables provide all of the essential nutrients for life. They are alive and filled with water. They are great in a salad and make refreshing juices. Their wide variety adds color and flavor to grains, soups, pastas and pizzas. In addition, they are extremely helpful in creating a "Snowbeing"...

Artichokes

Steamed Artichokes with Lemon Herb Dressing

2 artichokes
Water
Lemon herb dressing

Steam artichokes for 20-30 minutes. Serve with lemon herb dressing.

Asparagus

Sautéed Asparagus

1 bunch asparagus
1 tablespoon olive oil
or 2 ounces of water
2-4 garlic cloves
Fresh ground pepper to taste
Bragg's to taste
Lemon (optional)

> **Asparagus bottoms** tend to be hard and filled with fiber. Either peel the bottoms with a vegetable peeler or cut them off (approximately 1 inch).

Rinse asparagus and peel or cut off bottoms. Pour olive oil or water in pan. Use medium to high heat depending on your pan. Press garlic in oil. Add asparagus and sauté to desired texture (5-10 minutes). Season with Bragg's and fresh ground pepper. You're ready to serve.

Steamed Asparagus

1 bunch asparagus
Water

Rinse asparagus and peel or cut off bottoms. Steam asparagus until desired texture (5-10 minutes). Serve with dressing of your choice.

Broccoli

Broccoli Sautéed with Garlic

½ broccoli
1 tablespoon olive oil
or 2 ounces of water
2-4 garlic cloves
1 teaspoon arrow root powder
mixed in 2 ounces of water(optional)
Fresh ground pepper to taste
Bragg's to taste

Rinse broccoli and peel or cut off bottoms. Pour olive oil or water in pan. Use medium to high heat depending on your pan. Press garlic in oil. Add broccoli and sauté to desired texture (5-10 minutes). Season with Bragg's and fresh ground pepper. If you want a thicker sauce, mix 1 teaspoon of arrow root powder with 2 ounces of water, then add to sauté for the last 30 seconds You're ready to serve.

Steamed Broccoli

½ broccoli
Water

> **Steaming vegetables in a pot without a steamer tray** has saved me on more than one occasion. When I can't find my steamer tray or do not have one, I fill the bottom of a pot with an inch of water. Then place the vegetables in the pot and bring the water to a boil. The vegetables steam fine without the tray.

Rinse broccoli and peel or cut off bottoms. Steam broccoli until desired texture (5-10 minutes). Serve with dressing of your choice.

Cabbage

Stuffed Cabbage Rolls

4-6 cabbage leaves
Water
Vegetable stir fry (see vegetable sautés)
¼ cup chopped cilantro

Steam cabbage leaves, roll them up with vegetable stir fry and chill in refrigerator. Serve with fresh cilantro.

Carrots

Carrot juice (see Vegetable Juices)

Carrot Sticks

Carrots

Peel carrots with a vegetable peeler, cut off tops and cut into sticks.

Carrots in bean, grain, soup, vegetable and stir fry, dishes...

Steamed Carrots

Carrots
Water

Rinse or peel carrots and cut off tops. Cut carrots in desired shape. Steam carrots until desired texture (7-15 minutes). Serve with dressing of your choice.

Celery

Celery Sticks

Celery

Rinse celery, cut off tops and cut into sticks.

Enjoy celery in bean, grain, soup, vegetable and stir fry dishes...

Collards

Collard Greens sautéed with Sesame Seeds

1 bunch collards
Raw sesame seeds (optional)
1 tablespoon olive oil
or 2 ounces of water
2-4 garlic cloves
Fresh ground pepper to taste
Bragg's to taste

Rinse collard greens. Pour olive oil or water in pan. Use medium to high heat depending on your pan. Press garlic in oil. Add collard greens and sauté to desired texture (2-4 minutes). Sprinkle sesame seeds in pan and sauté for the last minute. Season with Bragg's and fresh ground pepper. You're ready to serve.

Steamed Collard Greens

1 bunch collard greens
Water

Rinse, cut and steam collard greens until desired texture (4-7 minutes). Serve with dressing of your choice.

Corn

Creamed Corn

3-4 ears corn
½ garlic cloves
Fresh ground pepper to taste
Bragg's to taste

Steam or roast corn. Remove corn kernels from cob. Purée ingredients in food processor and serve.

Roasted Corn or Steamed Corn

2-4 ears corn
Water

Roast corn in oven with husks on bake at 400 degrees until desired texture (15-25 minutes). To steam corn, peel corn then steam corn until desired texture (4-7 minutes).

Eggplant

Baba Kanouj

2-3 eggplants
4 ounces soaked sesame seeds
2-4 garlic cloves
½ teaspoon cumin and paprika
Fresh ground pepper to taste
Bragg's to taste

Bake whole eggplant for 25-35 minutes on 400 degrees. Then peel and purée in food processor. Blend soaked sesame seeds with garlic in a blender with enough of the soaked water to make a thick, creamy consistency. Purée baked eggplant and thick, creamy sesame seed paste in food processor and serve.

Baked Eggplant Slices

2-3 eggplants
½ teaspoon olive oil
½ teaspoon cumin
½ teaspoon paprika
Fresh ground pepper to taste
Bragg's to taste

Rinse eggplant and cut into approximately ½ inch circular slices. Put a thin coat of olive oil (½ teaspoon or less) or use vegetable oil spray on a baking sheet. Put eggplant slices on sheet and season with Bragg's and spices. Then bake for 25-40 minutes on 400 degrees. If you want this dish seasoned more - halfway through baking flip eggplant slices and season other side, then resume baking. If you want to make this dish faster. Broil both sides of eggplant first. Then bake for 10-20 minutes. The former takes less watching.

Baked Eggplant Slices with Red Pepper Sauce

2-3 eggplants
½ teaspoon olive oil
½ teaspoon cumin
½ teaspoon paprika
Fresh ground pepper to taste
Bragg's to taste

Red pepper sauce (see Sauces for ingredients)

Rinse eggplant and cut into approximately ½ inch circular slices. Put a thin coat of olive oil (½ teaspoon or less) or use vegetable oil spray on a baking sheet. Put eggplant slices on sheet and season with Bragg's and spices. Then bake for 25-40 minutes on 400 degrees. If you want this dish seasoned more - halfway through baking flip eggplant slices and season other side, then resume baking. If you want to make this dish faster. Broil both sides of eggplant first. Then bake for 10-20 minutes. The former takes less watching.

While eggplant is baking... chop up onion, purée 1 red pepper in food processor and dice or slice the rest of the red peppers. Peel and press garlic into wok style frying pan with olive oil or water. Cook on medium to high heat. Add onion and red pepper. Sauté until aldanté. Then add red pepper purée and lower temperature to simmer. Cook until baked eggplant is finished. Then serve baked eggplant on plate with red pepper sauce and a touch of parsley for special effects.

Curried Eggplant

2-3 eggplants
1 onion
2-4 garlic cloves
1 tablespoon olive oil
½ teaspoon thyme and mint leaves
¼ cup chopped parsley
2 tablespoons of curry powder
1 teaspoon arrow root powder
4-6 ounces of water
Fresh ground pepper to taste
Bragg's to taste

Peel and dice eggplant. Sauté with chopped onion and pressed garlic. Use 2-4 ounces of water to keep eggplant from sticking. Add herbs and spices when eggplant softens. Then mix arrow root powder with 2 ounces of water and add for the last 30 seconds of sauté.

Eggplant Paté

2-3 eggplants
1-2 garlic cloves
½ teaspoon olive oil
½ teaspoon cumin and paprika
Fresh ground pepper to taste
Bragg's to taste

Bake whole eggplant for 25-35 minutes on 400 degrees. Then peel and purée in food processor with garlic, herbs spices and oil. You are ready to serve.

Garlic

Baked Garlic

1-2 garlic bulbs
½-1 teaspoon olive oil (optional)

Bake garlic in oven on sheet on 400 degrees for 15-25 minutes.

Green Beans

Sautéed String Beans with Garlic

16 ounces green beans
2-3garlic cloves
1 tablespoon olive oil
Fresh ground pepper to taste
Bragg's to taste

Rinse string beans. Pour olive oil or water in pan. Use medium to high
heat depending on your pan. Press garlic in pan. Add string beans and
sauté to desired texture (5-8 minutes). Sprinkle sesame seeds in for the
last minute of sauté. Season with Bragg's and fresh ground pepper.
You're ready to serve.

Spicy Thai String Beans

16 ounces green beans
½ onion
2-3 garlic cloves
1 tablespoon olive oil
Fresh ground pepper to taste
Bragg's to taste
1 teaspoon Thai spices
2 tablespoons sesame seeds (optional)

Rinse string beans. Pour olive oil or water in pan. Use medium to high heat depending on your pan. Press garlic in pan. Add string beans and sauté to desired texture (5-8 minutes). Sprinkle sesame seeds in for the last minute of sauté. Season with Bragg's, Thai spices and fresh ground pepper. You're ready to serve.

Steamed String Beans

16 ounces string beans
Water

Rinse and steam string beans until desired texture (5-10 minutes).

Jerusalem artichokes

Jerusalem Artichokes with Lemon Herb Sauce

16 ounces Jerusalem artichokes
Water
Lemon herb dressing

Rinse and steam Jerusalem artichokes until desired texture (10-15 minutes). Serve with lemon herb dressing on side for dipping.

Lettuce

Bib
Boston
Butter
Green leaf
Red leaf
Red oak
Red romaine
Romaine

Lettuce is versatile. I use lettuce in the following: Shredded in food processor served with sprouts and grains or beans. Rolled up with paté, vegetables, beans, grains or nut & seed creations. Guacamole served on romaine leaves...and especially salads!

Mushrooms

Grilled Portabello

2-3 Portabello mushrooms
1 teaspoon olive oil
1 table spoon chopped parsley
½ teaspoon thyme
½ teaspoon cumin and paprika
Fresh ground pepper to taste
Bragg's to taste

> **Wipe dirt off mushrooms with a paper towel.** Try not to rinse. This will keep the mushrooms' flavor concentrated.

Put a thin coat of olive oil (½ teaspoon or less) or use vegetable oil spray on a baking sheet. Put Portabello mushroom caps on sheet and season with Bragg's and spices. Then grill for 20-30 minutes on 400 degrees.

Mushroom Gravy

4-6 ounces soaked cashews
1 teaspoon arrow root powder
16 ounces of mushrooms
½ onion
1-2 garlic cloves
1 teaspoon olive oil
1 tablespoon chopped parsley
½ teaspoon thyme
Fresh ground pepper to taste
Bragg's to taste

Pour olive oil or water in pan. Press garlic in pan. Cut up onion and sauté with pressed garlic for a couple of minutes (until onion is soft and/or clear) on medium to high heat depending on your pan. Add Mushrooms and sauté to desired texture (5-8 minutes). Blend soaked cashews with a teaspoon of arrow root powder, Bragg's and fresh ground pepper into a cream in blender. Add blended cashew cream to mushrooms and onion and stir on low heat until desired consistency. You're ready to use.

Mushroom Paté (cooked)

4-6 ounces soaked cashews
16 ounces of mushrooms
½ onion
1-2 garlic cloves
1 teaspoon olive oil
1 tablespoon chopped parsley
½ teaspoon thyme
Fresh ground pepper to taste
Bragg's to taste

Sauté onion, garlic and mushrooms with olive oil. Put herbs and spices in for the last minute of cooking. Purée soaked cashews in food processor or run through champion juicer with blank screen. Then purée sauté with cashews and add raw mushrooms for consistency.

Mushroom Paté (uncooked)

4-6 ounces soaked cashews
16 ounces of mushrooms
¼ onion
½-1 garlic clove
1 tablespoon chopped parsley
½ teaspoon thyme
Fresh ground pepper to taste
Bragg's to taste

Purée soaked cashews in food processor or run through champion juicer with blank screen. Then purée cashews, raw mushrooms, onion, garlic, herbs and spices.

Sautéed Mushrooms

16 ounces of mushrooms
2-3 garlic cloves
1 tablespoon olive oil
1 tablespoon chopped parsley
½ teaspoon thyme
Fresh ground pepper to taste
Bragg's to taste

Wipe dirt off mushrooms. (Try not to rinse. This will keep the mushrooms' flavor concentrated.) Pour olive oil or water in pan. Use medium to high heat depending on your pan. Press garlic in pan. Add mushrooms and sauté to desired texture (5-8 minutes). Season with Bragg's and fresh ground pepper. You're ready to serve.

Sautéed Mushrooms and Onions

16 ounces of mushrooms
½ onion
2-3 garlic cloves
1 tablespoon olive oil
1 tablespoon chopped parsley
½ teaspoon thyme
Fresh ground pepper to taste
Bragg's to taste

Wipe dirt off mushrooms. (Try not to rinse. This will keep the mushrooms' flavor concentrated.) Pour olive oil or water in pan. Press garlic in pan. Cut up onion and sauté with pressed garlic for a couple of minutes (until onion is soft and/or clear) on medium to high heat depending on your pan. Add mushrooms and sauté to desired texture (5-8 minutes).

Sautéed Portabello

2-3 Portabello mushrooms
½ onion
2-3 garlic cloves
1 tablespoon olive oil
¼ cup chopped parsley
½ teaspoon thyme
Fresh ground pepper to taste
Bragg's to taste

Wipe dirt off mushrooms. (Try not to rinse. This will keep the mushrooms' flavor concentrated.) Pour olive oil or water in pan. Press garlic in pan. Cut up onion and sauté with pressed garlic for a couple of minutes (until onion is soft and/or clear) on medium to high heat depending on your pan. Place mushroom caps over onion and garlic and turn heat down to simmer. Cover with top (5-10 minutes).

Onions

Sautéed Onions

1-2 onions
2-3 garlic cloves
1 tablespoon olive oil
1 tablespoon chopped parsley
½ teaspoon thyme
Fresh ground pepper to taste
Bragg's to taste

Pour olive oil or water in pan. Press garlic in pan. Cut up onions and sauté with pressed garlic and spices until desired texture on medium to high heat, depending on your pan.

Peas

Steamed Peas with Mashed Potatoes

12- 16 ounces peas
Water
Mashed potatoes (see potatoes)

Steam peas, remove from pod and serve with mashed potatoes.

Peppers

Sautéed Peppers

2-3 peppers
½ onion
2-3 garlic cloves
1 tablespoon olive oil
¼ cup chopped parsley
½ teaspoon thyme
Fresh ground pepper to taste
Bragg's to taste

Pour olive oil or water in pan. Press garlic in pan. Slice peppers and sauté with pressed garlic and spices until desired texture on medium to high heat depending on your pan.

Stuffed Roasted Peppers with Millet

Peppers
Millet (see grains)

Put a thin coat of olive oil (½ teaspoon or less) or use vegetable oil spray on a baking sheet. Bake whole peppers for 20-30 minutes on 400 degrees. Stuff peppers with millet.

Steamed Peppers Stuffed with Quinoa

Peppers
Quinoa (see Grains)
Red Pepper Sauce (see Sauces)

Steam peppers for 4-6 minutes until desired texture. Then stuff with **quinoa** (see Grains) and serve with **red pepper sauce** (see Sauces).

Potatoes

Baked Potatoes

Potatoes

Can be eaten plain, with sautéed vegetables, with sauces, in salads, rolled in lettuce leaves, even on sandwiches or pizzas...

Rinse potatoes and scrub clean with a vegetable brush. Bake potatoes on 400 degrees for 45-60 minutes depending on size and texture of choice.

Bake potatoes on oven rack. Potatoes contain much more moisture and flavor by not puncturing them!

Baked Potato Chips

Potatoes

Rinse potatoes and scrub clean with a vegetable brush. Thinly slice potatoes and place on a lightly oiled baking sheet. Bake on 350-400 degrees for 20-30 minutes. Remember to flip them. A food processor with a slicing attachment is quick, easy and provides uniform slices.

Mashed Potatoes

3-5 potatoes (16-24 ounces)
1-2 garlic cloves
1 teaspoon olive oil
1 tablespoon chopped parsley
¼ teaspoon thyme
Fresh ground pepper to taste
Bragg's to taste

Rinse potatoes and scrub clean with a vegetable brush. Cut potatoes into chunks and boil for 10-15 minutes. Put garlic and herbs in food processor and chop finely. Add potatoes, olive oil, Bragg's, pepper and some of the boiled water from the potatoes and purée.

Potato Pancakes

3-5 potatoes (16-24 ounces)
½ onion
1-2 garlic cloves
1 teaspoon olive oil
1 tablespoon chopped parsley
¼ teaspoon thyme
¼ teaspoon cumin
¼ teaspoon paprika
¼ teaspoon cayenne (optional)
Fresh ground pepper to taste
Bragg's to taste

Rinse potatoes and scrub clean with a vegetable brush. Finely dice garlic and onion in food processor. Sauté garlic and onion with olive oil in pan. Grate potatoes in food processor. Add potatoes and spices to sauté. Form potatoes into a pancake. Brown each side. You can easily flip your pancake by sliding it onto a plate then turning the plate over the pan. You may have to flip the pancake a few times. Then slide the pancake onto a lightly oiled baking pan and bake on 350-400 degrees for 30-40 minutes until desired texture.

Steamed Potatoes

Potatoes

Rinse potatoes and scrub clean with a vegetable brush. Slice potatoes and steam for 15-20 minutes depending on thickness of your slices.

Spinach

Sautéed Spinach

1 bunch spinach
2-3 garlic cloves
1 tablespoon olive oil
¼ teaspoon thyme
Fresh ground pepper to taste
Bragg's to taste

Rinse spinach and dry in a salad spinner. Cut spinach into salad size. Press garlic into pan with olive oil. Sauté spinach with spices on medium to high heat for about 2-3 minutes.

Squash

Sautéed Squash

2-4 squash (16-24 ounces)
2-3 garlic cloves
1 tablespoon olive oil
¼ teaspoon thyme
Fresh ground pepper to taste
Bragg's to taste

Clean squash with vegetable brush. Slice squash into strips and sauté in pan with olive oil, garlic and spices for 5-10 minutes.

Sautéed Squash and Onion

2-4 squash (16 ounces)
½ onion
2-3 garlic cloves
1 tablespoon olive oil
¼ teaspoon thyme
Fresh ground pepper to taste
Bragg's to taste

Clean squash with vegetable brush. Cut onion into thin strips. Slice squash into strips and sauté in pan with olive oil, garlic, onion and spices for 5-10 minutes.

Steamed Squash

Squash

Clean squash with vegetable brush. Slice squash and steam between 5-10 minutes depending on desired texture.

Sweet Potatoes or yams

Baked Sweet Potato

Sweet potatoes or yams

Clean sweet potatoes with vegetable brush and bake on 400 degrees for 50-70 minutes depending on size.

Baked Sweet Potato Chips

Sweet potatoes or yams

Clean sweet potatoes with vegetable brush. Thinly slice sweet potatoes with food processor and bake on 350 degrees for 25-35 minutes depending on size and thickness.

Mashed Sweet Potatoes

Sweet potatoes or yams
Garlic
Olive oil
Bragg's

Clean sweet potatoes with vegetable brush. Cut sweet potatoes into chunks and boil for 15-20 minutes. Purée sweet potatoes with a touch of garlic, olive oil, spices and some sweet potato water in a food processor.

Sweet Potato Pie

2-4 sweet potatoes or yams
12 ounces flour from whole grain wheatberries
 or use whole wheat flour
1½ ounces olive oil
1 tablespoon cinnamon
1 teaspoon vanilla
2-3 ounces hot water
¼ teaspoon Bragg's

Clean sweet potatoes with vegetable brush and bake on 400 degrees for 50-70 minutes depending on size. Grind up wheatberries with grinder into flour. Add cinnamon and baking powder to flour. Add olive oil and vanilla to water, then mix with flour to form crust. Form crust in pie shell. Remove skin from baked sweet potatoes and purée in food processor. Put purée in pie shell and bake on 350 for 30-40 minutes.

Vegetable Sauté or Stir Fry

Your choice of vegetables (asparagus, broccoli, cabbage, carrots, celery, mushrooms, onion, spinach...)
Olive oil or water
Garlic
Hers and spices of choice
Fresh ground pepper to taste
Bragg's to taste

Sauté or stir fry your favorite vegetables with spices, herbs, garlic and olive oil or water. Add fresh ground pepper and Bragg's to taste.

Zucchini

Sautéed Zucchini with Garlic

1-3 zucchinis (16 ounces)
½ onion (optional)
2-3 garlic cloves
1 tablespoon olive oil
¼ teaspoon thyme
2-4 ounces water to keep zucchini
from sticking to pan
Sesame seeds (optional)
Fresh ground pepper to taste
Bragg's to taste

Clean zucchini with vegetable brush. Cut zucchini into thin strips and sauté in pan with olive oil, garlic, onion and spices for 5-10 minutes. Add sesame seeds for the last minute of cooking.

Steamed Zucchini

Zucchini

Clean zucchini with vegetable brush. Slice zucchini and steam between 5-10 minutes, depending on desired texture.

Grains

Grains can be sprouted or cooked. They are versatile and can be prepared and eaten in many creative ways. Grains provide substance and are great to soak up the delightful flavors of vegetables, sauces and dressings. Their compact, condensed and power packed structure releases consistent and continuous energy throughout the day. I like to mix and match grains with sauces and vegetables. Feel free to be creative. That's what I do!

Brown Rice

8 ounces brown rice
16 ounces water

Put brown rice and water in a pot. Bring to a boil, then lower heat to low or warm and cook for 40 minutes. Turn off heat and let rice sit for 20 minutes until you are ready to serve.

Brown Rice Loaf

8 ounces brown rice
4-6 ounces soaked cashews
2 carrots
1 stem celery
¼-½ onion
4 ounces of mushrooms
1 tablespoon olive oil
2-3 garlic cloves
¼ cup chopped parsley
¼ teaspoon thyme and/or oregano
2-3 leaves sage
Fresh ground pepper to taste
Bragg's to taste

Put brown rice and water in a pot. Bring to a boil, then lower heat to low or warm and cook for 40 minutes. Turn off heat and let rice sit for 20 minutes until you are ready to serve.

Chop carrots, celery, onion, mushrooms and herbs in food processor. Blend soaked cashews with Bragg's, garlic and pepper into thick cream. Mix rice, chopped vegetables and cashew cream together and form into a loaf in a lightly oiled bread or casserole dish. Cover with lid or foil and bake for an hour on 350 degrees.

Brown Rice Sushi

8 ounces cooked brown rice
4-6 sheets Nori
Wasabi
Vegetables **(asparagus, cucumber, carrot, spinach, string beans, mushrooms...)**
1 avocado
Scallions
Lemon for dipping
Bragg's for dipping

Put brown rice and water in a pot. Bring to a boil, then lower heat to low or warm and cook for 40 minutes. Turn off heat and let rice sit for 20 minutes until you are ready to serve.

Roll brown rice, steamed or sautéed vegetables, avocado, scallions and cucumber in nori. Slice into bite size pieces and serve with wasabi, lemon and Bragg's.

Brown Rice with Sautéed Mushrooms

Brown rice
Sautéed mushrooms (see Vegetables)

Put brown rice and water in a pot. Bring to a boil, then lower heat to low or warm and cook for 40 minutes. Turn off heat and let rice sit for 20 minutes until you are ready to serve. Serve with sautéed mushrooms.

Grain Loaf

8 ounces brown rice
4 ounces millet
4 ounces quinoa
4 ounces lentils (optional)
4-6 ounces soaked cashews
2 carrots
1 stem celery
2-3 garlic cloves
¼-½ onion
4 ounces of mushrooms
1 tablespoon olive oil
¼ cup chopped parsley
¼ teaspoon thyme and/or oregano
2-3 leaves sage
Fresh ground pepper to taste
Bragg's to taste

Put brown rice and water in a pot. Bring to a boil, then lower heat to low or warm and cook for 40 minutes. Turn off heat and let rice sit for 20 minutes until you are ready to serve.

Put millet and water in a pot. Bring to a boil, then lower heat to low or warm and cook for 25 minutes. Turn off heat and let millet sit until you are ready to serve.

Put quinoa and water in a pot. Bring to a boil, then lower heat to low or warm and cook for 20 minutes. Turn off heat and let quinoa sit until you are ready to serve.

Grind lentils into flour with grinder and add warm water to form lentil paste.

Chop carrots, celery, onion, mushrooms and herbs in food processor. Blend soaked cashews with Bragg's, garlic and pepper into thick cream. Mix grains, lentil paste, chopped vegetables and cashew cream together and form into a loaf in a lightly oiled bread or casserole dish. Cover with lid or foil and bake for an hour on 350 degrees.

Millet

8 ounces millet
16 ounces water
1 red pepper
¼-½ onion
1 teaspoon olive oil
1-2 garlic cloves
¼ cup chopped parsley
¼ teaspoon thyme and/or oregano
Fresh ground pepper to taste
Bragg's to taste

Put millet and water in a pot. Bring to a boil then simmer on low or warm for 25 minutes. Turn off heat and let millet sit until you are ready to use.

Chop vegetables, herbs and spices together in a food processor and mix with millet in pot. Cover millet mixture and let sit until you are ready to serve.

Oatmeal

8 ounces oats
16-24 ounces water
1 teaspoon vanilla
1 tablespoon cinnamon (to taste)

Put oats and water in a pot. Bring to a boil then lower heat to low or warm and stir for 5 minutes. You're ready to serve!

Popcorn

Air popped popcorn

If popcorn doesn't pop properly, it might have dried out. Try storing it in the refrigerator for a couple of days to absorb moisture.

Sometimes I spray Bragg's and sprinkle paprika on air popped popcorn.

Quinoa with Onions and Herbs

8 ounces quinoa
16 ounces water
1 red pepper
¼-½ onion
1 teaspoon olive oil
1-2 garlic cloves
¼ cup chopped parsley
¼ teaspoon thyme and/or oregano
Bragg's to taste
Fresh ground pepper to taste

Put quinoa and water in a pot. Bring to a boil, then lower heat to low or warm and cook for 20 minutes. Turn off heat and let rice sit until you are ready to serve. Chop vegetables, mushrooms, herbs and spices together in a food processor and mix with quinoa, olive oil and Bragg's in pot. Cover quinoa mixture and let sit until you are ready to serve.

Quinoa with Scallions and Herbs

8 ounces quinoa
16 ounces water
1 red pepper
¼ cup chopped scallions
1 teaspoon olive oil
1-2 garlic cloves
¼ cup chopped parsley
¼ teaspoon thyme and/or oregano
Fresh ground pepper to taste
Bragg's to taste

Put quinoa and water in a pot. Bring to a boil the lower heat to simmer, low or warm for 20 minutes. Turn off heat and let quinoa sit until you are ready to use. Chop scallions, herbs and spices together in a food processor and mix with quinoa, olive oil and Bragg's in pot. Cover quinoa mixture and let sit until you are ready to serve.

Tabouleh

8 ounces bulgar (cracked) wheat
8-12 ounces boiling water
1 red pepper
¼-½ onion
1 teaspoon olive oil
1-2 garlic cloves
¼ cup chopped parsley
¼ teaspoon thyme and/or oregano
Bragg's to taste
Fresh ground pepper to taste

Pour wheat into boiling water and remove from heat. Cover wheat with a kitchen towel for 40 -60 minutes until chewy. Pour off water by straining wheat through a strainer. Chop vegetables, herbs and spices together in a food processor and mix with wheat, olive oil and Bragg's in dish. Cover wheat mixture and cool in refrigerator until you are ready to serve.

Waffles

Use any mixture of the following grains to make flour:
(wheatberries, oats, quinoa, millet, brown rice)
1½ cups grain flour
8-10 ounces water
1 teaspoon vanilla
1 tablespoon cinnamon
1 teaspoon olive oil
½ teaspoon baking powder
Maple syrup
Raw almond, cashew
or macadamia butter (optional)

Waffles are treats. Treats are foods I make on occasion. They are great for holidays or down time. They are warm, filling and remind me of my childhood. I use them sparingly, I guess that is why they remain treats.

Grind grains into flour with grinder and mix with cinnamon and baking powder. Mix water and vanilla. Pour liquid and oil into flour mixture and stir with fork until smooth. Pour batter onto heated waffle iron. Serve with maple syrup and raw nut butter.

Whole Wheat Pie Shell

12 ounces flour from whole grain wheatberries
or use whole wheat flour
1½ ounces olive oil
1 tablespoon cinnamon
1 teaspoon vanilla
2-3 ounces hot water
¼ teaspoon Bragg's

Grind wheat into flour and mix with cinnamon. Mix water, Bragg's and vanilla. Pour liquid and oil into flour and mix lightly. Round dough into ball and form pie shell in pie dish.

Whole Wheat Stuffing

½ whole wheat bread (16 ounces)
4-8 ounces chestnuts (optional)
1 red pepper
¼-½ onion
2 carrots
1 stem celery
8 ounces of mushrooms
1 teaspoon olive oil
1-2 garlic cloves
¼ cup chopped parsley
¼ teaspoon thyme and/or oregano
Fresh ground pepper to taste
Bragg's to taste

Dry bread crumbs soak up the juices and flavors of the sauté and make a mouth watering stuffing. If bread crumbs are still moist, put them on a baking sheet and bake on 350 degrees until they are dry.

Bake or boil chestnuts for 15-20 minutes. Then remove from shell. Bake or toast whole wheat slices until dark brown and crispy. Then let cool and harden on rack. Shred vegetables, mushrooms in food processor and sauté with garlic, chestnuts and olive oil. Put herbs and spices in for the last minute of sauté. Chop toast into bread crumbs in food processor. Mix bread crumbs with sauté, and serve!

Nuts & Seeds

Nuts and seeds contain the blueprints to grow into plants and trees. Their amazing energy is awakened by soaking in water and absorbing sunlight. The high fat, carbohydrate and protein content are broken down into essential fatty acids, sugars and amino acids. When I soak raw nuts and seeds before I eat them, I feel more energy and have better digestion.

Note: Soak nuts and seeds for 8 hours before use!

Nuts & Seeds

Almonds
Brazil nuts
Cashews
Filberts (Hazelnuts)
Macadamia nuts
Pecans
Pine nuts
Pistachios
Pumpkin seeds
Sesame seeds
Sunflower seeds
Walnuts

> **Raw unprocessed Nuts & Seeds are alive.** Soaking them releases natural living energy. Soaking awakens the seed of life from hibernation. The nuts and seeds start the germination process and begin to break down into amino acids, carbohydrates and fatty acids. Soaking makes nuts and seeds easier to digest and assimilate. Thereby giving you more energy.

Nut & Seed Butters

Soaked nuts or seeds

Run soaked nuts or seeds (soak for 8 hours in twice the amount of water) through champion juicer with blank "screen." Serve on bread, toast, crackers, celery, cucumbers, peppers, rolled up in romaine leaves... Almond butter is one of my favorites!

Nut & Seed Cheeses

8 ounces soaked nuts or seeds
½-1 clove garlic
¼ cup finely chopped parsley
¼ teaspoon thyme and/or oregano
Fresh herbs to taste
Fresh ground pepper to taste
Bragg's to taste

Run soaked nuts or seeds through champion juicer with blank "screen." Mix nut or seed paste with herbs and spices. Pack paste tightly and shape in a round cheese form. Cover to keep moisture in. Chill and serve.

Nut & Seed Dips

8 ounces soaked nuts or seeds
½-1 clove garlic
¼ cup chopped parsley
¼ teaspoon thyme and/or oregano
Fresh herbs to taste
Fresh ground pepper to taste
Bragg's to taste

Soak nuts or seeds for 8 hours with twice as much water. Blend soaked nuts or seeds to desired consistency by adding soaking water gradually. Then blend in herbs and spices. Chill and serve with celery sticks, cucumbers, peppers, romaine leaves, crackers, potato chips, baked potatoes, steamed vegetables...Cashew and sesame seed dips are my favorite!

Nut & Seed Milks

Soaked nuts or seeds

Soak nuts or seeds for 8 hours with twice as much water. Blend with enough of soaking nut water for desired consistency and strain. Use for a quick energy drink, with oatmeal, or other grain cereals. Almond and cashew milk are my favorite!

Soaked Nuts & Seeds

Choose one of the above nuts or seeds and soak for 8 hours. Then munch away. You can have them for snacks, in salads or use them for nut & seed cheeses, butters, dips and milks.

Peas & Beans

Peas and beans make great sprouts. They are wonderful in stews or salads. I love them served over shredded lettuce and sprouts. They make great soups and add substance to vegetables, grains and pastas. They are hearty and provide continuous and consistent energy throughout the day.

Note: Soak peas and beans for 8 hours before use!

Anasazi Beans

16 ounces soaked anasazi beans
1-2 peppers
(red, yellow or green)
1 onion
4-8 garlic cloves
¼ cup cilantro
¼ cup chopped parsley
1 tablespoon of leaves
Thyme or oregano
¼ cup basil
and other herbs (optional)
2-4 cups water for
desired consistency
Fresh ground pepper to taste
Bragg's to taste

Raw unprocessed peas & beans are hibernating. Soaking them releases natural living energy. Soaking awakens the seed of life from hibernation. The beans start the germination process and begin to break down into amino acids, carbohydrates and fatty acids. Soaking makes beans easier to digest and assimilate, thereby giving you more energy.

Soak beans with 3 times as much water overnight for 8 hours. In the morning, place chopped ingredients and water in crockpot on high. In 8 hours your meal is ready to be served. For added color, add ¼ cup chopped peppers. If you want a creamy spread, then purée beans in food processor or blender.

Black Beans

16 ounces soaked black beans
1-2 peppers (red, yellow or green)
1 onion
4-8 garlic cloves
¼ cup cilantro
¼ cup chopped parsley
1 teaspoon thyme or oregano leaves
¼ cup basil and other herbs (optional)
2-4 cups water for desired consistency
Fresh ground pepper to taste

Bragg's to taste

Soak beans with 3 times as much water overnight for 8 hours. In the morning, place chopped or diced ingredients in crockpot with water on high. In 8 hours your meal is ready to be served. For added color add ¼ cup chopped peppers to bowl of soup. If you want a creamy spread, then purée beans in food processor or blender.

Black-Eyed Peas

16 ounces soaked black-eyed peas
1 onion
4-8 cloves of garlic
¼ cup chopped parsley
1 teaspoon thyme or oregano leaves
2-4 cups water for desired consistency
Fresh ground pepper to taste
Bragg's to taste

Soak black eyed peas with 3 times as much water overnight for 8 hours. In the morning, place chopped or diced ingredients in crockpot with water on high. In 8 hours your meal is ready to be served. For added color add ¼ cup chopped peppers to bowl of soup. If you want a creamy spread, then purée beans in food processor or blender.

Creamy Chickpea Curry Spread

16 ounces soaked garbanzo beans
1 onion
2-3 carrots
2-3 stems celery
4-8 garlic cloves
¼ cup cut up parsley
Curry spices
1 teaspoon thyme or oregano leaves
2-4 cups water for desired consistency
Fresh ground pepper to taste
Bragg's to taste

Soak beans with 3 times as much water overnight for 8 hours. In the morning, place chopped or diced ingredients in crockpot with water on high. In 8 hours your meal is ready to be served. Add curry spices for flavor. Purée beans in food processor.

Garbanzo Beans

16 ounces soaked garbanzo beans
1 onion
2-3 carrots
2-3 stems celery
4-8 cloves garlic
¼ cup cut up parsley
1 teaspoon thyme or oregano leaves
2-4 cups water for desired consistency
Fresh ground pepper to taste
Bragg's to taste

Soak beans with 3 times as much water overnight for 8 hours. In the morning, place chopped or diced ingredients in crockpot with water on high. In 8 hours your meal is ready to be served. If you want a creamy spread, then purée beans in food processor or blender.

Hummous

16 ounces soaked garbanzo beans
4-8 garlic cloves
¼ cup chopped parsley
1 teaspoon thyme or oregano leaves
2-4 cups water for desired consistency
½ teaspoon cumin and paprika
Fresh ground pepper to taste
Bragg's to taste

Soak beans with 3 times as much water overnight for 8 hours. In the morning, place chopped or diced ingredients in crockpot with water on high. In 8 hours your beans should be a thick paste. Blend soaked sesame seeds in blender into a thick cream. Then mix with garbanzo paste in food processor.

Great Northern Beans

16 ounces soaked great northern beans
1 onion
2-3 carrots
2-3 stems celery
4-8 garlic cloves
¼ cup chopped parsley
1 teaspoon thyme or oregano leaves
2-4 cups water for desired consistency
Fresh ground pepper to taste
Bragg's to taste

Soak beans with 3 times as much water overnight for 8 hours. In the morning, place chopped or diced ingredients in crockpot with water on high. In 8 hours your meal is ready to be served. For added color add ¼ cup chopped peppers to bowl of soup. If you want a creamy spread, then purée beans in food processor or blender.

Lentils (green, red, yellow)

16 ounces soaked lentils
1 onion
2-3 carrots
2-3 stems celery
4-8 garlic cloves
¼ cup chopped parsley
1 teaspoon thyme or oregano leaves
2-4 cups water for desired consistency
Fresh ground pepper to taste
Bragg's to taste

Soak lentils with 3 times as much water overnight for 8 hours. In the morning, place chopped or diced ingredients in crockpot with water on high. In 8 hours your meal is ready to be served. If you want a creamy spread, then purée lentils in food processor or blender. Some Indian restaurants Dahl.

Lima Beans

16 ounces soaked lima beans
1 onion
2-3 carrots
2-3 stems celery
4-8 garlic cloves
¼ cup chopped parsley
1 teaspoon thyme or oregano leaves
2-4 cups water for desired consistency
Fresh ground pepper to taste
Bragg's to taste

Soak lima beans with 3 times as much water overnight for 8 hours. In the morning, place chopped or diced ingredients in crockpot with water on high. In 8 hours your meal is ready to be served. If you want a creamy spread, then purée lima beans in food processor or blender.

Navy Beans

16 ounces soaked navy beans
1 onion
2-3 carrots
2-3 stems celery
4-8 garlic cloves
¼ cup chopped parsley
1 teaspoon thyme or oregano leaves
2-4 cups water for desired consistency
Fresh ground pepper to taste
Bragg's to taste

Soak navy beans with 3 times as much water overnight for 8 hours. In the morning, place chopped or diced ingredients in crockpot with water on high. In 8 hours your meal is ready to be served. For added color add ¼ cup chopped peppers to bowl of soup. If you want a creamy spread, then purée navy beans in food processor or blender.

Pinto Beans

16 ounces soaked pinto beans
1-2 peppers (red, yellow or green)
1 onion
4-8 garlic cloves
¼ cup cilantro
¼ cup chopped parsley
1 teaspoon thyme or oregano leaves
2-4 cups water for desired consistency
Fresh ground pepper to taste
Bragg's to taste

Soak pinto beans with 3 times as much water overnight for 8 hours. In the morning, place chopped or diced ingredients in crockpot with water on high. In 8 hours your meal is ready to be served. For added color add ¼ cup chopped peppers to bowl of soup. If you want a creamy spread, then purée pinto beans in food processor or blender.

Pastas

Pastas are fun and simple to make. They come in a wide variety of shapes, sizes and flavors. I like fresh pastas with herbs whenever they are available. Pastas soak up flavor like grains and are great for a quick meal. Also, they promote conversation and romance...

I love putting on some music, dimming the lights, lighting candles and embarking on an intimate pasta adventure♥

Pasta

Dry or fresh pasta with no eggs.

Angel hair
Buckwheat noodles
Fetuccini
Linguini
Penne
Spaghetti
Ziti

Pastas are quick and simple to make. Boil some water and cook for 3-10 minutes depending on your pasta. Rinse with water. Then mix with your favorite sauce from my sauce section.

Sauces

Sauces spice up grains, vegetables, pastas, and pizzas. They add flavor, color and aroma making plain foods tantalizing meals. Here are some of my favorite mouthwatering sauces...

Alfredo Sauce

6-8 ounces cashews
½-1 garlic clove
1 teaspoon parsley for garnish
¼ teaspoon thyme and/or oregano
Fresh ground pepper to taste
Bragg's to taste

Blend, you're done.

Eggplant Topping

Baked eggplant (see Vegetables)

Cut up seasoned baked eggplant and you are ready to mix with the dish of your choice.

Garbanzo Bean Topping

Cooked garbanzo beans (see Peas & Beans)

Serve beans with your favorite pasta.

Garlic Sauce

6-8 ounces soaked nuts or seeds
½-1 garlic clove
½ teaspoon parsley for garnish
¼ teaspoon thyme and/or oregano
Fresh ground pepper to taste
Bragg's to taste

Blend, you're done.

Garlic/Broccoli Sauce

½ steamed broccoli (16 ounces)
½-1 garlic clove
1 tablespoon chopped Parsley
¼ teaspoon thyme and/or oregano
Fresh ground pepper to taste
Bragg's to taste

Chop herbs and spices in food processor. Add steamed broccoli to herbs and spices and chop.

Herb Sauce

½-1 garlic clove
¼ cup chopped parsley
¼ teaspoon thyme and/or oregano
¼ cup chopped basil
1-2 tablespoon olive oil
Fresh ground pepper to taste
Bragg's to taste

Chop herbs in food processor and mix with ½-1 tablespoon of olive oil over each dish.

Mushroom Sauce

Portabello, shitake, oyster, button, or your choice

Sautéed mushrooms (see Vegetables)

Sauté mushrooms and serve with your favorite pasta.

Pesto

4-6 ounces soaked pine nuts
½-1 garlic clove
¼-½ cup chopped basil (1 bunch)
¼ cup parsley
¼ teaspoon thyme and/or oregano
Fresh ground pepper to taste
Bragg's to taste

Chop herbs in food processor with pine nuts or purée into a creamy paste and serve.

Red Pepper Sauce

2-3 red peppers
½ onion
2-3 garlic cloves
1 tablespoon olive oil
¼ cup chopped parsley
½ teaspoon thyme
Fresh ground pepper to taste
Bragg's to taste

Pour olive oil or water in pan. Press garlic in pan. Cut up onion, dice or slice half of the peppers and sauté both with pressed garlic and spices. Purée other half of peppers in food processor. Pour pepper purée in sauté and simmer for 20 minutes.

Salsa

2-4 tomatoes
¼-½ onion
2-3 garlic cloves
¼ cup chopped cilantro
1 tablespoon chopped parsley
¼ teaspoon thyme
½ lemon (juice)
½-1 jalepeño (optional)
¼ teaspoon cayenne
Fresh ground pepper to taste
Bragg's to taste

> If you use jalepeño peppers you can lessen the fire by removing some of the seeds.

Chop onions and herbs in food processor. Dice tomatoes and mix with chopped onions, herbs, Bragg's, lemon and spices.

Spinach Topping with side of Zucchini

Spinach and zucchini
(see Vegetables for ingredients)

Clean zucchini with vegetable brush. Rinse spinach and dry in a salad spinner. Cut up spinach. Cut zucchini into thin strips and sauté in pan with olive oil, garlic and spices for 5-10 minutes. Put zucchini on plate and sauté spinach in the zucchini juices with garlic and spices for 2-3 minutes. Mix spinach with grain or pasta of choice and serve on side of zucchini.

Sautéed Zucchini

Sautéed zucchini **(see Vegetables for ingredients)**

Clean zucchini with vegetable brush. Slice onions into thin strips. Cut zucchini into thin strips and sauté in pan with olive oil, garlic, onions and spices for 5-10 minutes.

Vegetable Curry

1 pepper
2 carrots
1 stem celery
¼ broccoli
¼ eggplant
8 ounces of mushrooms
¼-½ onion
2-3 garlic cloves
1 tablespoon olive oil
1 tablespoon chopped parsley
½ teaspoon thyme
Curry spices to taste
Fresh ground pepper to taste
Bragg's to taste

Chop up or shred vegetables. Sauté with herbs and curry spices.

Vegetable Thai

1 pepper
2 carrots
1 stem celery
¼ broccoli
¼ eggplant
8 ounces of mushrooms
¼-½ onion
2-3 garlic cloves
1 tablespoon olive oil
1 table spoon chopped parsley
½ teaspoon thyme
Thai spices to taste
Fresh ground pepper to taste
Bragg's to taste

Chop up or shred vegetables. Sauté with herbs and Thai spices.

Pizzas

Pizzas are fun, simple and quick. They go great with soups, salads, pastas or on their own. There are unlimited creations. Here are a few of my favorites.

Pizzas

> **I eat whole wheat pizzas on occasion.** I keep them to a minimum because I find processed foods and bread products tend to make me sluggish!

Pizza Crusts

Frozen whole wheat or sour dough pizza crust. If you are really ambitious, make your own!

Garlic/Red Pepper Pizza Topping

2-3 red peppers
½ onion
3-5 garlic cloves
1 tablespoon olive oil
¼ cup chopped parsley
½ teaspoon thyme
Fresh ground pepper to taste
Bragg's to taste

Pour olive oil or water in pan. Press garlic in oil. Cut up onion, slice peppers and sauté with pressed garlic and spices until desired texture on medium to high heat depending on your pan. Put topping on pizza crust and bake for 10-15 minutes or until desired texture.

Eggplant Pizza Topping

Baked or sautéed eggplant (see vegetables)

Put topping on pizza crust and bake for 10-15 minutes or until desired texture.

Mushroom/Onion Pizza Topping

16 ounces of mushrooms
½ onion
3-5 garlic cloves
1 tablespoon olive oil
1 tablespoon chopped parsley
½ teaspoon thyme
Fresh ground pepper to taste
Bragg's to taste

Wipe dirt off mushrooms. (Try not to rinse. This way you will keep the mushrooms' flavor concentrated.) Pour olive oil or water in pan. Press garlic in pan. Cut up onion and sauté with pressed garlic for a couple of minutes (until onion is soft and/or clear) on medium to high heat depending on your pan. Add mushrooms and sauté to desired texture (5-8 minutes). Put topping on pizza crust and bake for 10-15 minutes, or until desired texture.

Spinach/Garlic Pizza Topping

1 bunch spinach
3-5 garlic cloves
1 tablespoon olive oil
¼ teaspoon thyme
Fresh ground pepper to taste
Bragg's to taste

Rinse spinach and dry in a salad spinner. Cut spinach into salad size. Press garlic into pan with olive oil. Sauté spinach with spices on medium to high heat for about 2-3 minutes. Put topping on pizza crust and bake for 10-15 minutes, or until desired texture.

Vegetable Curry Pizza Topping

1 pepper
2 carrots
1 stem celery
¼ broccoli
¼ eggplant
8 ounces of mushrooms
¼-½ onion
2-3 garlic cloves
1 tablespoon olive oil
1 tablespoon chopped parsley
½ teaspoon thyme
Curry spices to taste
Fresh ground pepper to taste
Bragg's to taste

Chop up or shred vegetables (in food processor) and sauté with herbs and curry spices. Put topping on pizza crust and bake for 10-15 minutes or until desired texture.

Burritos & Roll Ups

> I eat whole wheat tortillas on occasion.
> I keep them to a minimum because I find
> processed foods and bread products tend
> to make me sluggish!

Burritos

Beans (choose any of the following beans:
            anasazi, black, garbanzo, kidney, pinto...)
Brown rice
Sautéed vegetables
Spinach
Lettuce
Sprouts
Guacamole
Salsa
Whole wheat tortillas

Choose your favorite beans and fill a whole wheat tortilla with any or all
of the above ingredients. If the burrito is huge (ranchero style), then
serve on a plate with silverware. If you can roll it up, pick it up and
enjoy! If you want to avoid bread, eat this over shredded lettuce or
sprouts.

Roll Ups

Take the beans of your choice and purée in food processor. Take any or
all of the above ingredients and roll them up in a whole wheat tortilla. If
you want to avoid the bread, eat this over shredded lettuce or
sprouts....or try lettuce roll-ups!

One of my favorites is a creamy curried chickpea roll up

Fun Feasts

Delight your palate with an all American Holiday Feast. Then take your taste buds to India, Italy, Japan, Mexico, the Middle East and Thailand. You will have dining experiences to savor and remember!

Holiday Feast

Roasted corn, cranberry sauce, grain or brown rice loaf, green beans, mashed potatoes, mushroom gravy, stuffing, sweet potato pie

Indian Feast

Curry cucumber salad, creamy curry chickpea soup, sautéed curried vegetables with brown rice, puréed lentil paste (Dahl)

Italian Feast

Garbanzo bean soup, Italian salad, fetuccini pasta with sautéed spinach and a side of zucchini, garlic/red pepper pizza

Japanese Feast

Miso soup with buckwheat noodles, miso salad, nori rolls, vegetable stir fry with brown rice

Mexican Feast

Mexican salad, creamy black bean soup, burritos, guacamole, rice, salsa, corn chips

Middle Eastern Feast

Garden salad with tahini dressing, vegetable soup, baba kanouj, hummous, cucumber slices, olives, pita

Thai Feast

Spicy Thai cucumber salad, vegetable soup with Thai spices, Thai stir fry with brown rice

Seasonal Menus

Seasonal menus are weekly menus with a full day of meals for a week in Spring, Summer, Fall and Winter. I buy whatever is in season, abundant, good quality and economical. I included these menus to give you a guide for creating weekly menus and buying weekly ingredients. Feel free to follow, augment or change them. Most importantly enjoy what Mother Nature has to offer and let NoBrainer Nutrition empower you!

Spring Menus

Day 1/ Spring

Morning (Fruits)

♦ Orange juice

Mid morning (Fruits)

♦ Pineapple/papaya smoothie

Late morning (Fruits)

♦ Papaya salad

Afternoon (Vegetables, Grains, Legumes, Beans, Nuts & Seeds)

♦ Carrot/celery/cucumber juice

Mid afternoon

♦ Avocado garden salad

Late afternoon

♦ Fetuccini with spinach and a side of sautéed zucchini

Evening

♦ Vegetable juice

Mid evening

♦ Tea

Day 2/ Spring

Morning (Fruits)

♦ Orange juice

Mid morning (Fruits)

♦ Papaya/pineapple/avocado fruit salad

Late morning (Fruits)

♦ Orange/papaya smoothie

Afternoon (Vegetables, Grains, Legumes, Beans, Nuts & Seeds)

♦ Carrot/celery/beet juice

Mid afternoon

♦ Asparagus salad

Late afternoon

♦ Vegetable juice

Evening

♦ Vegetable curry with brown rice

Mid evening

♦ Tea

Day 3/ Spring

Morning (Fruits)

◆ Orange juice

Mid morning (Fruits)

◆ Papaya/pineapple salad

Late morning (Fruits)

◆ Orange/pineapple juice

Afternoon (Vegetables, Grains, Legumes, Beans, Nuts & Seeds)

◆ Carrot/lettuce/cucumber juice

Mid afternoon

◆ Mashed potatoes with sautéed mushrooms and onions

Late afternoon

◆ Vegetable juice

Evening

◆ Romaine salad with creamy garlic dressing and steamed artichokes

Mid evening

◆ Vegetable juice

Day 4/ Spring

Morning (Fruits)

♦ Pineapple juice

Mid morning (Fruits)

♦ Sliced mango

Late morning (Fruits)

♦ Orange juice

Afternoon (Vegetables, Grains, Legumes, Beans, Nuts & Seeds)

♦ Carrot/cucumber juice

Mid afternoon

♦ Baked potato

Late afternoon

♦ Vegetable juice

Evening

♦ Spinach salad with avocado tomato basil dressing

Mid evening

♦ Tea

Day 5/ Spring

Morning (Fruits)

♦ Orange/papaya smoothie

Mid morning (Fruits)

♦ Orange juice

Late morning (Fruits)

♦ Mango pie

Afternoon (Vegetables, Grains, Legumes, Beans, Nuts & Seeds)

♦ Carrot/celery juice

Mid afternoon

♦ Gazpacho soup

Late afternoon

♦ Vegetable juice

Evening

♦ Burritos

Mid evening

♦ Tea

Day 6/ Spring

Morning (Fruits)

◆ Papaya smoothie

Mid morning (Fruits)

◆ Mango/pineapple salad

Late morning (Fruits)

◆ Orange juice

Afternoon (Vegetables, Grains, Legumes, Beans, Nuts & Seeds)

◆ Carrot juice

Mid afternoon

◆ Potato pancakes

Late afternoon

◆ Vegetable juice

Evening

◆ Brown rice with sautéed mushrooms

Mid evening

◆ Tea

Day 7/ Spring

Morning (Fruits)

♦ Orange juice

Mid morning (Fruits)

♦ Papaya/mango/banana salad

Late morning (Fruits)

♦ Orange/papaya juice

Afternoon (Vegetables, Grains, Legumes, Beans, Nuts & Seeds)

♦ Carrot/spinach juice

Mid afternoon

♦ Guacamole with cucumber slices, celery sticks and romaine leaves

Late afternoon

♦ Vegetable juice

Evening

♦ Vegetable soup

Mid evening

♦ Tea

Weekly Ingredients/ Spring

Produce

Artichokes
Asparagus
Avocados
Banana
Lemon
Oranges
Mangos
Papayas
Pineapples
Tomatoes
Carrots
Celery
Cucumbers
Garlic
Mushrooms
Onions
Potatoes
Romaine
Spinach
Sprouts
Zucchini

Herbs

Basil

Cilantro
Dill
Oregano
Parsley
Thyme

Spices

Basil
Bragg's
Cayenne
Cumin
Curry powder
Dill
Paprika
Pepper corns

Dry goods

Barley
Brown Rice
Cashews
Fetuccini or pasta of choice
Split peas
Tea
Tortillas for burritos

Summer Menus

Day 1/ Summer

Morning (Fruits)

- Cantaloupe juice

Mid morning (Fruits)

- Honeydew salad

Late morning (Fruits)

- Peach juice

Afternoon (Vegetables, Grains, Legumes, Beans, Nuts & Seeds)

- Carrot/celery/cucumber juice

Mid afternoon

- Miso garden salad

Late afternoon

- Quinoa with a side of sautéed zucchini

Evening

- Vegetable juice

Mid evening

- Tea

Day 2/ Summer

Morning (Fruits)

♦ Peach juice

Mid morning (Fruits)

♦ Peach/grape/banana fruit salad

Late morning (Fruits)

♦ Banana/grape smoothie

Afternoon (Vegetables, Grains, Legumes, Beans, Nuts & Seeds)

♦ Carrot/celery/beet juice

Mid afternoon

♦ Cucumber salad

Late afternoon

♦ Vegetable juice

Evening

♦ Brown rice with vegetable Thai sauté

Mid evening

♦ Tea

Day 3/ Summer

Morning (Fruits)

♦ Watermelon juice

Mid morning (Fruits)

♦ Papaya/banana/raisin fruit salad

Late morning (Fruits)

♦ Peaches

Afternoon (Vegetables, Grains, Legumes, Beans, Nuts & Seeds)

♦ Carrot/lettuce/cucumber juice

Mid afternoon

♦ Brown rice with sautéed broccoli

Late afternoon

♦ Vegetable juice

Evening

♦ Romaine with tomato basil dressing

Mid evening

♦ Vegetable juice

Day 4/ Summer

Morning (Fruits)

♦ Nectarine juice

Mid morning (Fruits)

♦ Cherries

Late morning (Fruits)

♦ Peach pie

Afternoon (Vegetables, Grains, Legumes, Beans, Nuts & Seeds)

♦ Carrot/cucumber juice

Mid afternoon

♦ Baked potato with steamed zucchini and creamy garlic sauce

Late afternoon

♦ Vegetable juice

Evening

♦ Spinach salad with mushrooms and lemon herb dressing

Mid evening

♦ Tea

Day 5/ Summer

Morning (Fruits)

♦ Grape juice

Mid morning (Fruits)

♦ Nectarines

Late morning (Fruits)

♦ Plums

Afternoon (Vegetables, Grains, Legumes, Beans, Nuts & Seeds)

♦ Carrot/celery juice

Mid afternoon

♦ Gazpacho soup with avocado chunks

Late afternoon

♦ Vegetable juice

Evening

♦ Nori Rolls with Miso Soup

Mid evening

♦ Tea

Day 6/ Summer

Morning (Fruits)

- Plum juice

Mid morning (Fruits)

- Banana coconut cream pie

Late morning (Fruits)

- Papaya juice

Afternoon (Vegetables, Grains, Legumes, Beans, Nuts & Seeds)

- Carrot juice

Mid afternoon

- Colorful garden salad with avocado/tomato dressing

Late afternoon

- Vegetable juice

Evening

- Chickpea curry roll ups

Mid evening

- Tea

Day 7/ Summer

Morning (Fruits)

♦ Apricot juice

Mid morning (Fruits)

♦ Bananas

Late morning (Fruits)

♦ Grapes

Afternoon (Vegetables, Grains, Legumes, Beans, Nuts & Seeds)

♦ Carrot/spinach juice

Mid afternoon

♦ Avocado salad

Late afternoon

♦ Vegetable juice

Evening

♦ Black bean soup

Mid evening

♦ Tea

Weekly Ingredients/ Summer

Produce

Apricots
Avocados
Bananas
Beets
Cantaloupe
Cherries
Coconut
Grapes
Honeydew
Mangos
Nectarines
Papayas
Peaches
Plums
Tomatoes
Watermelon
Carrots
Celery
Cucumbers
Garlic
Mushrooms
Onions
Potatoes
Romaine
Spinach
Sprouts
Zucchini

Herbs

Basil
Dill
Oregano
Parsley
Thyme

Spices

Basil
Bragg's
Cayenne
Cumin
Curry powder
Dill
Miso
Paprika
Pepper corns

Dry goods

Black beans
Brown rice
Cashews
Garbanzo beans
Penne or pasta of choice
Raisins
Tea
Tortillas for roll ups

Fall Menus

Day 1/ Fall

Morning (Fruits)

♦ Apple juice

Mid morning (Fruits)

♦ Apple/banana/date smoothie

Late morning (Fruits)

♦ Pears

Afternoon (Vegetables, Grains, Legumes, Beans, Nuts & Seeds)

♦ Carrot/celery/cucumber juice

Mid afternoon

♦ Mexican salad

Late afternoon

♦ Angel hair with pesto sauce

Evening

♦ Vegetable juice

Mid evening

♦ Tea

Day 2/ Fall

Morning (Fruits)

◆ Pear juice

Mid morning (Fruits)

◆ Apples

Late morning (Fruits)

◆ Banana/date smoothie

Afternoon (Vegetables, Grains, Legumes, Beans, Nuts & Seeds)

◆ Carrot/celery/beet juice

Mid afternoon

◆ Spicy Thai cucumber salad

Late afternoon

◆ Vegetable juice

Evening

◆ Quinoa with scallions and sautéed string beans

Mid evening

◆ Tea

Day 3/ Fall

Morning (Fruits)

♦ Orange juice

Mid morning (Fruits)

♦ Apple/grape juice

Late morning (Fruits)

♦ Banana/date/coconut fruit salad

Afternoon (Vegetables, Grains, Legumes, Beans, Nuts & Seeds)

♦ Carrot/lettuce/cucumber juice

Mid afternoon

♦ Millet with sautéed mushrooms and onions

Late afternoon

♦ Vegetable juice

Evening

♦ Black beans with brown rice

Mid evening

♦ Vegetable juice

Day 4/ Fall

Morning (Fruits)

♦ Grapes

Mid morning (Fruits)

♦ Apple/pear/banana/raisin fruit salad

Late morning (Fruits)

♦ Apple juice

Afternoon (Vegetables, Grains, Legumes, Beans, Nuts & Seeds)

♦ Carrot/cucumber juice

Mid afternoon

♦ Spinach salad with tomato basil dressing

Late afternoon

♦ Vegetable juice

Evening

♦ Ziti with garlic and broccoli sauce

Mid evening

♦ Tea

Day 5/ Fall

Morning (Fruits)

♦ Apple/banana/date smoothie

Mid morning (Fruits)

♦ Pears

Late morning (Fruits)

♦ Apple pie

Afternoon (Vegetables, Grains, Legumes, Beans, Nuts & Seeds)

♦ Carrot/celery juice

Mid afternoon

♦ Miso soup

Late afternoon

♦ Vegetable juice

Evening

♦ Brown rice with sautéed Portabello mushrooms

Mid evening

♦ Tea

Day 6/ Fall

Morning (Fruits)

♦ Orange/grapefruit juice

Mid morning (Fruits)

♦ Banana smoothie

Late morning (Fruits)

♦ Pear juice

Afternoon (Vegetables, Grains, Legumes, Beans, Nuts & Seeds)

♦ Carrot juice

Mid afternoon

♦ Baked eggplant

Late afternoon

♦ Vegetable juice

Evening

♦ Potato soup and salad

Mid evening

♦ Tea

Day 7/ Fall

Morning (Fruits)

♦ Apple/pear juice

Mid morning (Fruits)

♦ Bananas

Late morning (Fruits)

♦ Grapes

Afternoon (Vegetables, Grains, Legumes, Beans, Nuts & Seeds)

♦ Carrot/spinach juice

Mid afternoon

♦ Avocado soup with cucumbers

Late afternoon

♦ Vegetable juice

Evening

♦ Vegetable stir fry with brown rice

Mid evening

♦ Tea

Weekly Ingredients/ Fall

Produce

Apples
Avocados
Bananas
Dates
Grapes
Grapefruit
Lemon
Oranges
Pears
Tomatoes
Carrots
Celery
Cucumbers
Garlic
Mushrooms
Onions
Potatoes
Romaine
Sweet potatoes
Spinach
Sprouts
Zucchini

Herbs

Basil
Dill
Oregano
Parsley

Thyme

Spices

Basil
Bragg's
Cayenne
Cumin
Curry powder
Dill
Paprika
Pepper corns

Dry goods

Barley
Black beans
Brown Rice
Cashews
Split peas
Wheatberries
Tea
Tortillas
Ziti or pasta of choice

Winter Menus

Day 1/ Winter

Morning (Fruits)

♦ Orange juice

Mid morning (Fruits)

♦ Apples

Late morning (Fruits)

♦ Banana smoothie

Afternoon (Vegetables, Grains, Legumes, Beans, Nuts & Seeds)

♦ Carrot/celery/cucumber juice

Mid afternoon

♦ Quinoa with onion over chopped romaine

Late afternoon

♦ Garbanzo bean soup

Evening

♦ Vegetable juice

Mid evening

♦ Tea

Day 2/ Winter

Morning (Fruits)

♦ Orange/grapefruit juice

Mid morning (Fruits)

♦ Pears

Late morning (Fruits)

♦ Apple/banana/date smoothie

Afternoon (Vegetables, Grains, Legumes, Beans, Nuts & Seeds)

♦ Carrot/celery/beet juice

Mid afternoon

♦ Cream of broccoli soup

Late afternoon

♦ Vegetable juice

Evening

♦ Millet with vegetable curry

Mid evening

♦ Tea

Day 3/ Winter

Morning (Fruits)

♦ Grapefruit juice

Mid morning (Fruits)

♦ Apple/pear smoothie

Late morning (Fruits)

♦ Bananas

Afternoon (Vegetables, Grains, Legumes, Beans, Nuts & Seeds)

♦ Carrot/lettuce/cucumber

Mid afternoon

♦ Mashed sweet potatoes with sautéed broccoli

Late afternoon

♦ Vegetable juice

Evening

♦ Romaine lettuce & cucumber with creamy dill dressing

Mid evening

♦ Vegetable juice

Day 4/ Winter

Morning (Fruits)

♦ Apple juice

Mid morning (Fruits)

♦ Citrus salad

Late morning (Fruits)

♦ Pears

Afternoon (Vegetables, Grains, Legumes, Beans, Nuts & Seeds)

♦ Carrot/cucumber

Mid afternoon

♦ Baked sweet potato

Late afternoon

♦ Vegetable juice

Evening

♦ Lentil soup with rice

Mid evening

♦ Tea

Day 5/ Winter

Morning (Fruits)

♦ Pear juice

Mid morning (Fruits)

♦ Orange juice

Late morning (Fruits)

♦ Apple/pear/banana/raisin fruit salad

Afternoon (Vegetables, Grains, Legumes, Beans, Nuts & Seeds)

♦ Carrot/celery juice

Mid afternoon

♦ Pepper salad

Late afternoon

♦ Vegetable juice

Evening

♦ Pizza with sautéed mushroom and onions

Mid evening

♦ Tea

Day 6/ Winter

Morning (Fruits)

♦ Apple/banana/date smoothie

Mid morning (Fruits)

♦ Pear juice

Late morning (Fruits)

♦ Apple juice

Afternoon (Vegetables, Grains, Legumes, Beans, Nuts & Seeds)

♦ Carrot juice

Mid afternoon

♦ Cucumber with avocado chunks

Late afternoon

♦ Vegetable juice

Evening

♦ Curried chickpeas with brown rice and sautéed spinach

Mid evening

♦ Tea

Day 7/ Winter

Morning (Fruits)

♦ Orange juice

Mid morning (Fruits)

♦ Grapefruit juice

Late morning (Fruits)

♦ Apple juice

Afternoon (Vegetables, Grains, Legumes, Beans, Nuts & Seeds)

♦ Carrot/spinach juice

Mid afternoon

♦ Pizza with garlic and peppers

Late afternoon

♦ Vegetable juice

Evening

♦ Peppers stuffed with quinoa

Mid evening

♦ Tea

Weekly Ingredients/ Winter

Produce

Apples
Avocados
Bananas
Dates
Grapefruit
Lemon
Oranges
Pears
Carrots
Celery
Cucumbers
Garlic
Mushrooms
Onions
Potatoes
Romaine
Spinach
Sprouts
Sweet potatoes
Zucchini

Herbs

Basil

Dill
Oregano
Parsley
Thyme

Spices

Basil
Bragg's
Cayenne
Cumin
Curry powder
Dill
Paprika
Pepper corns

Dry goods

Barley
Brown Rice
Cashews
Fetuccini or pasta of
choice
Split peas
Tea
Tortillas

Index